# What experts are saying about

## *The End-of-Life Namaste Care Program for People with Dementia*
### *Second Edition*

"Everyone wins with the positive enveloping Namaste Care™ approach to advanced dementia—residential care providers, care teams, caring families and, best of all, people living with advanced dementia. Simard's wise, experienced, practical, rich, and detailed specifics interspersed with inspiring stories of small miracles make real and achievable all the abstract ideals of dignified, compassionate quality care."

—*Lisa P. Gwyther, MSW, LCSW, Co-author,* The Alzheimer's Action Plan, *Director, Duke Family Support Program, Duke University*

"Gives the reader a step-by-step guide to implementing this amazing program without incurring high labor cost or capital expense. The results of the Namaste Care™ program at EPOCH buildings have been nothing short of heartwarming and wonderful for all who are touched by it."

—*Joanna Cormac Burt, Chief Operating Officer, EPOCH Senior Living*

"The Namaste Care™ program revolutionizes how to lovingly provide care for those facing advanced dementia and empowers health care providers to find the person within using creative, multi-modal interventions. In her book, Joyce Simard leads you to the very heart of this approach to dementia care."

—*Russell Hilliard, PhD, LCSW, LCAT, MT-BC, CHRC, Vice President, Seasons Hospice & Palliative Care*

D08814820

# The End-of-Life

# *Namaste Care*™

## Program for People with Dementia

The End-of-Life

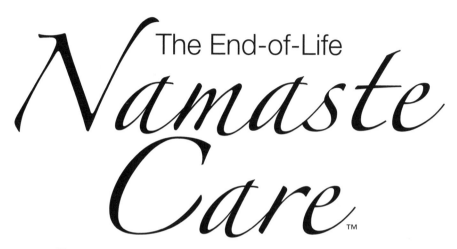

*Namaste Care*™

Program for People with Dementia

—SECOND EDITION—

Joyce Simard, M.S.W.

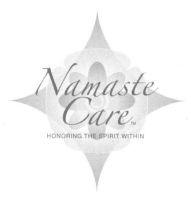

*Namaste Care*™

HONORING THE SPIRIT WITHIN

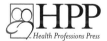

Baltimore • London • Sydney

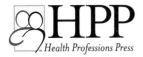

Health Professions Press, Inc.
Post Office Box 10624
Baltimore, Maryland 21285-0624

www.healthpropress.com

Interior, cover, and logo designs by Mindy Dunn.
Typeset by Barton Matheson Willse & Worthington, Baltimore, Maryland.
Manufactured in the United States of America by Versa Press, East Peoria, Illinois.

 Namaste Care™ and the Namaste Care logo are trademarks of
Health Professions Press, Inc.

The information provided in this book is in no way meant to substitute for a medical practitioner's advice or expert opinion. Readers should consult a medical practitioner if they are
interested in more information. This book is sold without warranties of any kind, express or
implied, and the publisher and author disclaim any liability, loss, or damage caused by the
contents of this book.

All of the case studies described in this book are based on the author's actual experiences, but
the names and identifying details have been changed to protect privacy. Exceptions include
Arden Courts of HCR ManorCare (throughout); EPOCH Senior Living (throughout); Seasons Hospice (Chapter 8); Vermont Veterans Home (pp. 45, 69); and Matthew and Celia Wilk
(throughout), whose stories recounted in this book are real and whose permission for this use
is gratefully acknowledged.

Library of Congress Cataloging-in-Publication Data

Simard, Joyce.
    The end-of-life Namaste Care program for people with dementia / by Joyce Simard. —
2nd ed.
        p. ; cm.
    Includes bibliographical references and index.
    ISBN 978-1-938870-02-6 (pbk.)
    I. Namaste Care (Program)  II. Title.
    [DNLM:  1. Alzheimer  Disease—nursing.  2. Dementia—nursing.  3. Holistic
Health.  4. Terminal Care—methods.  WY 152]
    RC521
    616.8'31029—dc23
                                                                    2013002144

British Library Cataloguing in Publication data are available from the British Library.

# Contents

# About the Author

**Joyce Simard, M.S.W.,** is a private geriatric consultant to skilled nursing centers, assisted living communities, and hospice organizations worldwide. She is also involved in research projects investigating the effects of Namaste Care™ in Australia and the United Kingdom. She earned her bachelor of arts in sociology and social work from Ithaca College in New York and her master's of social work from the University of Minnesota. She also serves as Adjunct Associate Professor at the School of Nursing and Midwifery, University of Western Sydney, Australia.

In addition to the Namaste Care program, Simard has developed other programs for people with memory loss. The Memory Enhancement Program (MEP) is for people experiencing memory loss above and beyond what is normal for their age and education. Residents in independent living and assisted living communities as well as those who participate in adult day programs benefit from this unique program. The Club is a program for residents in nursing facilities and assisted living who have moderate memory loss. Its implementation has resulted in a decrease in anti-psychotic medications as well as a decline in resident falls and improved staff and resident satisfaction.

Simard is the author of a children's book about aging and dementia, *The Magic Tape Recorder* (2007), which was published in several languages and is currently out of print.

Simard is an internationally recognized speaker who has presented both to families of people with dementia and to health care professionals in the United States, Europe, Australia, and parts of Asia. As a keynote or featured speaker at professional conferences, she is known for bringing humor and a light touch to serious subjects, teaching through stories of real experiences from her 35 years in health care. She also provides in-service training on a variety of subjects, including hospice, bereavement, comfort care, and activity programs for people with all stages of dementia.

More information can be found at www.joycesimard.com or www.namastecare.com, or by e-mailing joycesimard@earthlink.net.

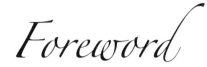

# Foreword

Publication of the first edition of *The End-of-Life Namaste Care Program for People with Dementia* encouraged many health care providers to reassess how to care for individuals with advanced dementia. Although Namaste Care™ was originally intended for implementation in long-term care facilities, the program has since been adapted in other settings where individuals with advanced dementia live, specifically assisted living communities and hospices. This second edition is a result of the expansion of Namaste Care and the popularity of the first edition.

Since the publication of the first edition, Namaste Care programs have been successfully implemented throughout the United States as well as in Australia, England, Scotland, and Greece. One large assisted living organization in the U.S., Arden Courts, chose to incorporate Namaste Care into all of its facilities. A hospice organization, Season's Hospice, is using the Namaste Care approach in all of its facilities as well, under its own customized name (Touch for All Seasons). The success of Namaste Care was also reflected in the selection of Joyce Simard, M.S.W., as one of *Provider* magazine's "20 to Watch" in 2013 for her compassion and commitment to providing quality of life at the end of life for individuals with advanced dementia.

Namaste Care is an enlightened program that strives to maintain the highest quality of life possible for individuals with severe and terminal dementia. This care involves the creation of a special room that provides a quiet, peaceful environment for residents in the last stage of the disease. Meaningful activities are individualized for each resident and a continuous presence of staff members provides both physical and sensory stimulation. Namaste Care does

not require additional staff, just some rethinking of staff assignments, and can be implemented with minimal programming cost.
This "high-touch" care can be taught to all staff as well as to family
members. The family members in particular appreciate the attention given to their loved ones.

I am sure that publication of this second edition of *The End-of-
Life Namaste Care Program for People with Dementia* will encourage
many more long-term care facilities, assisted living communities,
and hospices to pay greater attention to individuals with advanced
dementia as well as other terminal diseases and conditions. The
book will hopefully serve as an important road map in this effort
because it describes in detail how the program can be implemented,
how the Namaste Care team is established, how an appropriate
Namaste Care environment is created, and what the day's activities
could look like. In addition, the book discusses decision making
at the end of life and what is meant by "comfort care." An understanding of death and dying and the need for care after death are
also provided. Finally, the appendices include useful resources for
establishing a Namaste Care program.

Namaste Care provides residents and their families with quality care that addresses not only physical but also emotional and
spiritual needs. It reminds us that individuals with advanced dementia should not be isolated in their rooms, but instead need to live
their last days in a pleasant environment receiving loving care from
all staff and families.

*Ladislav Volicer, M.D., Ph.D., F.A.A.N., F.G.S.A.*
*Courtesy Full Professor, University of Southern Florida, School of Aging
    Studies, Tampa, Florida*
*Retired Clinical Director, Geriatric Research Education and Clinical
    Center (GRECC), Veterans Administration Hospital (Bedford,
    Massachusetts)*

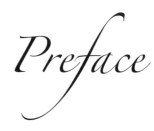

*Preface*

"I have lost myself."

AUGUSTE D.

On November 4, 1906, Dr. Alois Alzheimer gave a lecture in which he described Auguste D., a 51-year-old woman with symptoms of a progressive, cognitive impairment. He had been puzzled that a woman so young exhibited symptoms usually seen in those much older. After Auguste's death in April of 1906, Dr. Alzheimer performed an autopsy on her brain to try to determine the reason for her unusual behavior. When the brain samples were placed under a microscope, he discovered the plaques and neurofibrillary tangles that are now recognized as the markers of the disease that ultimately was named after this researcher: Alzheimer's disease. At the time, however, his lecture was virtually ignored by his colleagues and the material was deemed "not appropriate for a publication" (Maurer, Volk, & Gerbaldo, 1997).

More than a hundred years after this lecture, Dr. Alzheimer is internationally recognized as the physician who discovered Alzheimer's disease, a condition that at the beginning of the 21st century affects 5.4 million Americans and costs the U.S. health care system $200 billion per year (Alzheimer's Association, 2012). Alzheimer's is the sixth-leading cause of death and is second only to cancer as the most greatly feared disease among adults older than 55 (MetLife Foundation, 2011).

According to a quote taken from her medical records, Auguste D. cried out to Dr. Alzheimer, "I have lost myself." This lament is as relevant today to the millions of people struggling with Alzheimer's as it was to this woman a century ago. Another entry in Auguste's files quotes her husband as being upset with his wife's accusations of infidelity. Upsetting behavior such as this continues to distress present-day spouses, who are often bewildered by similar accusations. Unfortunately, the despair and confusion surrounding Alzheimer's continue.

Auguste D. was placed in a mental asylum. Today, thankfully, there are many more options to help family members care for people with Alzheimer's, including adult day services, home health care aides, housekeeping services, hospice, and respite care. This array of services provides support for the exhausting caregiving responsibilities that accompany Alzheimer's. The Alzheimer's Association reports that more than 60% of caregivers rate their emotional stress as very high and one-third report symptoms of distress (Alzheimer's Association, 2012).

If she lived today, perhaps Auguste's family would have been able to keep her at home for longer or maybe she would have resided in an assisted living community that specializes in the care of people with early and moderate dementia. When her dementia progressed to the point where she needed more care or her family could not afford for her to reside in an assisted living community, Auguste could have spent the last years of her life in a skilled nursing facility that offers a memory care neighborhood. Hospice services might have been available in the last days or months of her life, and bereavement services may have been offered to Auguste's husband after her death.

From diagnosis to death, family and professional care partners now have access to a variety of services and information on the psychosocial and medical needs and treatments to help make life easier for people with Alzheimer's. Books written by professionals, family members, and people with Alzheimer's are published on a regular basis. We know so much more about how people with Alzheimer's feel, how to help them live with the disease, and how to support their families.

Despite this increased attention, the experience of advanced dementia remains misunderstood and underserved, regardless if the person lives at home or in a long-term care setting or is receiving hospice services. The Alzheimer's Association has recommended that end-of-life care needs to be given more attention from researchers as well as health care practitioners (Alzheimer's Association, 2007). Nursing facilities tend to focus on medical care for residents with advanced dementia (i.e., monitoring vital signs and dispensing medication). Residents with advanced dementia are well groomed, changed, and fed. But what is their quality of life? The same can be said about residents in assisted living communities, as "aging in place" has increased the need for programming appropriate for people at each stage of dementia. Families are ill-informed of how to help their loved one in the final stages of the disease. A physician addressing hundreds of fellow physicians at an American Medical Directors conference said "without quality of life, quality of care doesn't matter that much." Namaste Care™ is all about quality of life.

In some nursing facilities, residents with advanced dementia are grouped around the nurses' station so that they can be observed. Other residents with advanced dementia are isolated in their rooms. Some nurses believe that the kindest way to care for residents with advanced dementia who are no longer ambulatory is to leave them in bed. These residents spend the rest of their lives in one room, alone for the majority of the day, their voices stilled by the disease. Because they can no longer cry out "I'm here" or "Help me," they are easy to forget in the busy life of a nursing facility. In some respects, they become invisible.

Since the first edition of this book was published, the number of residents in assisted living communities with advanced dementia has increased dramatically. Assisted living regulations are state specific and each state determines how physically and cognitively impaired a resident can be until he or she is moved to a nursing facility or the family is required to provide a private care assistant. In this second edition, I address the differences between nursing facilities and assisted living communities who are implementing Namaste Care. One chapter is devoted to the differences in these two long-term care settings.

*Rights.*

People with advanced dementia living in any care setting deserve the right to be acknowledged, enjoy meaningful activities, be in the presence of others, and receive the loving touch approach that is the foundation of Namaste Care. Richard Taylor eloquently reminds us in his insightful book *Alzheimer's From The Inside Out*: "I want and need to give and receive love. Even when I can't remember your name, will you please love me?" Namaste Care is all about giving and receiving love.

I developed the Namaste Care program to bring an improved quality of life to nursing facility residents in the last stages of Alzheimer's. Namaste (pronounced *nah-ma-stā*) is a Hindu term meaning "to honor the spirit within," a perfect name, I thought, for a program designed to acknowledge the person first, not the disease, and to honor the person in all aspects of his or her life. The Namaste Care program also removes the isolation surrounding many residents in health care settings and invites them to be in the presence of others in a place that is peaceful and filled with soft music, with the feeling of love surrounding them.

This book was written in the hope that you, the reader, will be inspired to enhance the care that is provided to residents, patients, family members, or clients with advanced dementia in whatever setting they call home. It also reflects a personal journey of mine of over 35 years in health care. My goal for writing this book was to provide easy-to-read, step-by-step advice on how to start a Namaste Care program in your organization or how to use Namaste Care approaches in a home setting. Vignettes of actual experiences are woven into each of the chapters as examples of how Namaste Care works. If you work in health care, you have no doubt experienced the humorous side of our work that makes a sometimes-difficult job less stressful. I hope that you will smile as you read about some of my less-than-stellar ideas and resident encounters.

When this book was first published, I never dreamed that Namaste Care would be used internationally. Programs now can be found in Australia, England, Scotland, and Greece. And those are just the ones I actually know exist.

I have changed some vocabulary in this second edition to reflect the ongoing shift in the United States from a medical model of care to a more compassionate, social, and person-centered model of care. I use *care partner* rather than *nursing assistant*. This new term shows how we need to help people with dementia continue to participate in their care for as long as possible. I also refer to the staff who work in a health care organization as *team members* to heighten the awareness that indeed it "takes a village" to provide quality care.

The people and organizations in this book are committed to providing a high quality of care. They are often the unsung heroes who go more than the extra mile for the residents they care for and care about. This book sings their praises and acknowledges their excellent work.

One such unsung hero is Lorna Reid, the education liaison nurse for ACCORD Hospice in Scotland. She has become a strong supporter of Namaste Care. Lorna once asked me to do a workshop for care homes and hospice staff. As the program ended, she read the following:

> "Do for one what you wish you could do for everyone." [quote from Andy Stanley, pastor, author, and founder of North Point Ministries, Inc.] I can't change the world on my own, but I can do for one what I wish I could do for everyone. In fact, that is the story of the hospice movement, which started with one nurse, turned social worker, turned physician, who encountered one patient. As the result of that encounter, she (Dame Cicely Saunders) set out on a journey to create a place where she could give to one group of people what she wished she could do for every group. One led to two which led to hundreds which led to thousands. And now hospice influences the care of people all over the world. So, I'm not going to let myself get overwhelmed. As long as I am able, I will keep on doing for one group what I wish I could do for every group. Maybe you will be encouraged to do the same.

And so, for as long as I am able, I too will not let myself get overwhelmed. I will offer to teach Namaste Care to one person or one group what I wish I could teach everyone. I will teach Namaste Care to people in one country what I wish I could teach people all over the world. And gradually I hope and I pray that the standards for quality of life for people with advanced dementia will improve.

Maybe you will be encouraged to do the same.

# Acknowledgments

The acknowledgments could easily be as long as the book. Many people, including residents, professional health care staff, and family members, have contributed to the formulation of Namaste Care™ over the years. A special thank you goes to Celia Wilk, wife of Matthew Wilk, who gave me permission to share how Namaste Care helped to fill her husband's last months and days with moments of joy. His death was, in fact, the motivation that led me to write this book.

Without support from the past and present administrators, department managers, and incredible staff of the Vermont Veterans Home (VVH), Namaste Care might still be an unrealized dream. The first Namaste Care program was up and running within 30 days of the administrator's, Earle Hollings, approval. It happened quickly because of the commitment of many dedicated individuals at VVH, especially Mary Longtin, who began providing Namaste Care before it had a name, and is one of those people who touches your life and leaves an indelible mark. Mary continues to be an inspiration to all whose lives she touches as she continues to be the lead Namaste Carer at VVH. Activity director Michele Burgess, dementia program director Christina Cosgrove, former director of nursing Marlene Restino, and charge nurse Jennie LaBrake and her team put a great deal of time and effort into getting the original Namaste Care program started. Although their Namaste Care program has changed over time, it is still thriving and provides special care to the veterans and their spouses who gave so much to the United States.

Under the dynamic leadership of COO Joanna Cormac-Burt and VP of clinical services Karen Roberts, EPOCH Senior Living has made a commitment to offer Namaste Care in each of their nursing facilities and will be offering the program in their new Bridges assisted living communities with memory care neighborhoods. They have raised the bar for providing quality care for residents with advanced dementia. Many of the excellent learning experiences in this book were made possible by the devotion and commitment of the leaders of EPOCH Senior Healthcare to provide excellent care for their residents through each stage of dementia. Thank you, all!

John J. Megara, the administrator at Hale Nani Rehabilitation and Nursing Center in Honolulu, Hawaii, is another strong supporter of Namaste Care and is helping to educate health care professionals about end-of-life care in that state. Mahalo, John.

For the past 4 years, I have been blessed to have worked with Russell Hilliard, national director of supportive care, Seasons Healthcare Management. Under his leadership, I was able to adapt Namaste Care for hospice patients with advanced dementia. Their unique program, called A Touch for All Seasons, has improved the quality of life for patients, their families, and the Seasons staff, an amazing group of people who are constantly seeking ways to improve end-of-life care. Seasons Hospice has sponsored me as a speaker on Namaste Care throughout the country as a service to the public. I have written a new chapter on the use of Namaste Care in hospice for this edition of the book that features my work with them. My life's work has been enriched by working with Seasons Hospice.

Thanks to a very special relationship with a unique assisted living company, Arden Courts Memory Care, I have written a chapter for this second edition on implementing Namaste Care in assisted living communities. With Pauline Coram, director of executive learning, leading the way and with the commitment of John Graham, VP and general manager of the assisted living division of HCR ManorCare, Arden Courts will be the first U.S. company to offer Namaste Care in all of their communities.

Namaste Care has also become internationally recognized as an innovative program of care for residents with advanced dementia. I am proud to have friends in the United Kingdom such as Arlette Beebeejaun, a home care manager at Exelcare who implemented the organization's first Namaste Care program. She has welcomed visitors from all over the U.K. and other European countries to learn from her staff how to implement Namaste Care and hear the benefits to their residents. Her regional director, Geraldine Finney, was great in helping me to understand some of the differences in the U.K. health care system.

Since publication of the first edition, I have been involved in two research projects. The first was with the University of Western Sydney, School of Nursing and Midwifery. Under the direction of Professor Esther Chang, project manager Michel Edenborough, and project officer Sara Karacsony, we were able to introduce Namaste Care in Australia. Lynn Mowbray, administrator at Minchinbury Manor, and Cate Good, administrator at Principal Shoalhaven, have developed wonderful Namaste Care programs and were very helpful to me as I included the Australian experience in this second edition.

The second research project is with St. Christopher's Hospice in London. A chance meeting in Lisbon, Portugal, with St. Christopher's chief executive, Dame Barbara Monroe, and Jo Hockley, nurse consultant and care home project and research team manager, resulted in funding a research project to look at outcomes of Namaste Care. Nurse researcher Min Stackpoole is leading this investigation.

This book would never have been written if not for the loving support of Ladislav Volicer. His cheerleading, methodical review of all chapters, and understanding of the medical issues that accompany dementia care were invaluable.

Finally, this book would never have reached so many health care professionals all over the world if Mary Magnus, director of publications for Health Professions Press, had not taken a chance on this unknown author, not once, but twice!

Thank you, Mary.

# CHAPTER 1

# The Beginning

I shall be telling this with a sigh
Somewhere ages and ages hence:
Two roads diverged in a wood, and I,
I took the one less traveled by,
And that has made all the difference.

ROBERT FROST

We never know how our lives will be shaped by events that initially seem insignificant but are actually profound turning points. My first interview for a social work position took place in Ithaca, New York, in 1978. Walking into a very old nursing facility, formerly a rehabilitation center for children with polio, I thought something like, "This is not for me; this will have to be a temporary position." All of the residents looked so old and disabled and sad. My adult life had revolved around children, four of my own and many foster babies. I believed that my social work career would focus on young people, perhaps foster care, something I knew about. I desperately wanted to make a difference. Children had a future; the elderly were at the end of their lives. As my peers rated social work jobs, the nursing home was not high on the list of sought-after positions. But as I have learned, sometimes the hard way, life has a way of leading you down the road less traveled.

As part of my interview, the administrator, Michael Apa, gave me a tour of the building. We walked around the first floor, when residents were being gathered for lunch. Mr. Apa asked me to help transport residents into the dining room; of course, I readily agreed.

My first efforts to move a wheelchair did not work. Tugging and then trying to lift it produced no forward movement. No one told me that wheelchairs have brakes. Needless to say, this new social worker had a lot to learn!

In spite of my ineptness, I was hired and began a career that would turn out to be my life's work, my mission, and my joy. The main responsibility in this position was admissions, keeping the beds full. Then, because of my eagerness to get to know residents and the lack of time in which to do it, I began to lead groups. I started with a group for residents' families, because I realized that many of them were struggling with feelings of guilt about placing their loved one in a nursing home. I also led a Discharge Planning Group for residents who were returning home and a Newcomers Group for newly admitted residents. Residents in my groups were alert, oriented, and able to express themselves, and I felt that my social work skills were being put to good use. Although we must have had residents with dementia, I do not remember working with them.

It was not until 1979, when our family was transferred to Minnesota, that my interest in residents with dementia surfaced. At Westwood Nursing Home in Saint Louis Park, Minnesota, I assumed responsibility for the dreaded second floor, where most of the residents had what we now know as Alzheimer's disease or a related dementia. At that time, residents were diagnosed with senile dementia, presenile dementia, or organic brain syndrome. Sometimes the medical records completely ignored their memory loss and just addressed the person's medical problems. Social workers did not enjoy working on the second floor because they could not use their counseling skills, and the nursing staff was frustrated when the residents did not listen or follow directions. In spite of being told not to go into other residents' rooms, they often did. Some wandered aimlessly or tried to leave the facility; occasionally they disrobed in public areas.

Because of this "bizarre" behavior (and yes, that is what we called behavior that we now know as symptoms of dementia), we placed these residents on the second floor. In fact, they were hidden from the tours we gave to families. No one wanted a prospective family to be frightened by seeing these residents and choose another nursing home.

We also thought that if we placed residents who were at risk for elopement on the second floor, they would be safer. As I recall, the doors leading to the stairs were alarmed, and most second floor residents could not figure out how to use the elevator, so the second floor seemed to be the best option for them.

Second floor residents were labeled as having behavioral problems or being combative. The solution was to medicate them "for their own good." When they were at risk of falling, we restrained them in geri-chairs. They would of course pound on the trays that restrained them in the chair and call out for help. So, to keep these residents quiet and "happy," we medicated them. If the medications did not work, we sent residents to the psychiatric unit of the local hospital. Of course they returned acting like zombies, with all the medication they had been given. I shudder when I look back on how well intentioned we were and how far we have come in knowing that medication is usually not the answer and that combativeness, now referred to as rejection of care, is usually caused by inappropriate approaches from care partners.

The nursing facility had a good reputation; we provided what was, at the time, good custodial care for residents with memory loss. They were kept changed, groomed, bathed, fed, and attended to medically. A few activity programs offered diversion in bits and pieces, but activity staff struggled to find ways to entertain residents with memory loss. Because they might act out during programs, they received fewer hours of dedicated activity services than other residents. The oriented residents appreciated being involved in activities and were very vocal that they wanted to be entertained and kept busy. They were simply more rewarding to work with. Clearly, we struggled with what to do with a group of residents who lived in another reality.

Counseling was impossible because of the residents' severe memory loss, so I thought that all my social work training was for naught. Nonetheless, as the director of the department, I let my staff choose where they wanted to work, and I ended up on the dreaded second floor. With little understanding of why a resident could not remember that her mother had died years ago or that she did not have to go home to care for her "children," who were now 50 years old, I was mystified about how to provide social work services to my residents.

All levels of staff were told to use reality orientation (RO) at all times. This approach taught us that it was important to constantly remind residents of their surroundings, the time, the place, the person, the truth. We believed that saying the same thing over and over would help residents with memory loss live in the present. When a resident asked where she was or said that she wanted to go home, we replied, "You are in a nursing home, your children are grown, and you do not need to fix dinner for them. Your children are adults with their own homes." Many residents looked for their mothers, and when we used RO and told them that their mother had died 20 years ago, they were devastated. This perpetually "new" information was shocking and upsetting to them. Here is a recollection of one of my first encounters with a resident who must have had Alzheimer's disease:

## SALLY

While I was getting to know residents on the second floor, a woman in her eighties approached me and asked whether I had seen her mother. My tender and compassionate response was that her mother had passed away. She, of course, was shocked at this information and dissolved into tears. Within 5 minutes, she approached me again with the same question. My response was the same: Her mother had died. Once again, she cried over the "recent" loss of her mother. This was quite demoralizing. After all, my job was to help the residents feel good, not cause them to cry. When Sally approached me the third time with the same question, my gut reaction was to try a different response. Not quite knowing what this line of questioning would produce, I asked her to describe her mother. With a big smile, she told me what her mother looked like and what a wonderful mother she was. We proceeded to have a delightful conversation about all kinds of things, and when our visit was over, I reassured her that I would look for her mother. The resident walked away very happy that someone would help her. Somehow my question, which had no basis in reality, reached this woman. At least for a moment, she was at peace.

## CHANGES IN DEMENTIA CARE

I decided that the best approach to working with residents on this floor was not to use RO. They needed a new tactic to help them live in their world, but what would that be? The answer came as a rather new and radical (at the time) change in how we cared for residents who had severe memory loss. A social worker named Naomi Feil (1982) introduced a new approach to replace RO, and she called it Validation Therapy. After attending one of her workshops, I could hardly contain my excitement. Someone was finally giving compassionate advice on how to work with residents who had memory loss and an altered sense of reality. The answer seemed to be to "join their journey," as my friend Kathy Laurenhue (www.wiser-now.com) teaches, rather than trying to drag them into our world. Validation Therapy offered us a simple way to help residents with memory loss live happier lives. Blanch is just one example of a resident who benefited from the shift from RO to Validation Therapy.

### *BLANCH*

> Blanch, a widow in her seventies with two grown sons and grandchildren, believed that she was on vacation and the nursing home was a hotel. Every morning she thanked the staff for the wonderful stay at the hotel but said her husband was picking her up so she could go home to care for her two small children. The staff hugged Blanch and told her how much they had enjoyed having her stay with them. Then they suggested that she have breakfast while waiting for her husband to arrive; after all, breakfast was already paid for! Blanch happily walked to the dining room, joined her friends for breakfast, and promptly forgot about going home. The next day it would all start again.

Years ago, Blanch would have been distressed each day as she was told the truth: that her husband was deceased, her sons were grown, and she was living in a nursing facility. Using the Validation Therapy approach, we supported Blanche in a way that helped her live a happier life, surrounded by friends in a great "hotel."

Another important change in dementia care for families and health care workers was the Alzheimer's Association. Founded in

1980, it emerged as the leading force in awakening the public's awareness of Alzheimer's disease. Beginning with a few family members and health care professionals, the association grew to become a respected organization with chapters throughout the United States. The Alzheimer's Association's mission is "to eliminate Alzheimer's disease through the advancement of research; to provide enhanced care and support for all affected; and to reduce the risk of dementia through the promotion of brain health." The association is dedicated to enhancing the quality of life of all people affected by Alzheimer's disease and related disorders through advocacy, education, and support systems while also promoting research efforts (Alzheimer's Association, 2012b).

As the number of people with Alzheimer's disease grew, so did the scope of services and programs offered by the Alzheimer's Association. They began to offer support groups not only for families but also for people with early Alzheimer's disease and for children whose lives were affected by grandparents with Alzheimer's disease. The association and most chapters offer conferences and other educational opportunities to help professionals working with people who have Alzheimer's disease.

In the 1980s interest in Alzheimer's disease grew as health care professionals realized that the number of residents in nursing facilities who had memory loss was significant and growing. They needed more information on how to treat and care for this special population. Articles on Alzheimer's disease started to appear in journals, and one journal was dedicated just to Alzheimer's disease. When I began my career, I rarely saw articles or books on Alzheimer's disease. Now, the pile of reading threatens to topple over when I get behind.

Researchers became aware that they needed to study a variety of care issues related to people with Alzheimer's disease and the burdens felt by their families. Alzheimer's disease became the hot topic of conversation for health care professionals. About this time drug companies began to sink millions of dollars into finding medications to help slow the progression and perhaps cure Alzheimer's disease. Public awareness of Alzheimer's disease increased dramatically in 1979 when Rita Hayworth made headlines announcing that she had Alzheimer's disease. This was followed 15 years later when Ronald Reagan also made his diagnosis public.

Nursing facilities providing care for the growing population of residents with dementia began to change as new approaches to caring for them began to emerge. Nursing facility owners realized that dementia care was a good business. Special care units (SCUs) emerged; these were secured areas within a facility that provided special activities for residents with dementia and special educational programs for staff. It was an exciting time as the long-term care industry explored ways to help residents with dementia maintain quality in their lives.

I was fortunate to be part of the new change in dementia care when, in 1990, I joined the Hillhaven Corporation, a leader in the care of residents with Alzheimer's disease. Under the leadership of Nancy Orr-Rainey, a department was created to develop SCUs (Orr-Rainey, 1994). These units were secured so residents would be in a safe, controlled environment. SCUs were designed with country kitchens so the women could feel at home, help prepare a meal, or sit at the kitchen table. Office spaces were established for men who had "work" to do. Secure outside courtyards were built so residents could enjoy being outside, planting gardens, or watching birds as they flocked around the bird feeders. Living rooms were arranged so that games could be played and families could visit in comfortable surroundings.

Nursing facilities realized that special dementia units were good for business. They recognized that SCUs with high-quality programming had healthy censuses, some with waiting lists. When the emergence of assisted living residences began to erode their private-pay census, many nursing facility companies found that a specialized dementia unit had the greatest potential to attract new private-pay residents. Most nursing facilities lose money on Medicaid residents; therefore, their ability to attract private-pay residents helps keep them solvent.

As more and more SCUs were developed, the need for a special activity program emerged. These residents needed something to do with their time. Most health care professionals agree that residents with moderate to advanced dementia rarely self-initiate meaningful

NAAP

activities and need continuous activity programming (Volicer, Simard, Pupa, Medrek, & Riordan, 2006). When a resident with dementia has nothing to do, he or she tends to engage in what are often called problem behaviors, such as wandering into other residents' rooms, going through others' belongings and taking items (I call them shoppers), or otherwise annoying other residents and their families.

One of my earliest experiences with a shopper was Joe. We knew he liked to wander into other residents' rooms, but what we did not know was that if he didn't have his dentures in his mouth, Joe would believe they were lost, and unbeknownst to us, he was on a quest to find them. When he died we were cleaning his bureau and discovered 15 pairs of dentures safely tucked away in the back of a drawer. This solved the mystery of the sudden rash of complaints we had been receiving about lost dentures.

I have found that residents like activities that remind them of earlier times in their lives. In fact, finding ways to keep residents involved in the life of the unit became my specialty. I discovered that some women like folding laundry or washing dishes. Mothers like rocking babies and folding baby clothes and cloth diapers. Men like having office work to do. We had cooking groups, sing-alongs, religious services, and exercise. The National Association of Activity Professionals (NAAP) emerged as a resource to help educate activity staff and increased awareness that activities were not just fun but therapeutically beneficial, especially for residents with Alzheimer's disease.

As nursing facilities grew more aware of the specialized needs of the residents with dementia, educational programs were offered to help staff understand how to provide care for residents with memory loss. Many training films and educational materials became available for health care professionals and family care partners. Today, basic Alzheimer's education is part of the orientation program in most nursing facilities and assisted living communities. Many states now mandate training in Alzheimer's disease for all staff.

Several years ago, the large nursing facility company that employed me as its national director of Alzheimer's services held a "Nursing Facility of the Future" meeting. When asked my thoughts on what the building should look like, I described creating a small, secured wing for the few oriented residents and devoting the rest of the building to people with various stages of memory loss. Everyone thought I was joking! Staff members in nursing facilities today say that at least 80% of residents who are not on the rehabilitation unit have some significant memory loss; it seems that I was ahead of my time with my prediction

Another change in dementia care took place in the 1990s when the assisted living industry began to realize that dementia care was a lucrative business. I was once again privileged to work with the Marriott Corporation and became their Alzheimer's specialist for Marriott Senior Living Services assisted living communities. I became immersed in every aspect of assisted living dementia care, from working with designers and choosing colors and fabrics to designing education programs for staff and activities for residents with early- and middle-stage Alzheimer's disease. Our units were created to be home-like surroundings that helped residents know what to do in a variety of spaces. We noticed that when the environment looked like a large home or a hotel, residents were less anxious and seemed more at home. They could identify the living room with its couches and television set, felt comfortable relaxing with other residents in the country kitchen, and clearly knew that the dining room was the place in which to eat. Marriott designed the dining rooms to look like restaurants. As a result, residents were on their best behavior, as they thought they were going out to eat. Many of the men insisted on receiving a check so they could fulfill their role of the male paying for the meal. We gave them a "check" and were often amused that a tip was added for the great service we provided!

## PHILOSOPHICAL CHANGES IN DEMENTIA CARE

With her Validation approach, Naomi Feil (1982) opened the door to a new way of caring for people with memory loss. Others have followed with a variety of approaches that continue to improve quality of life for people with dementia. Virginia Bell and David Troxel (1996, 2003) wrote about becoming a best friend to someone with Alzheimer's disease. Tom Kitwood's (1998) person-centered therapy recognizes the importance of the individual first,

Eden at Home          IDEAS

the disease second. Cameron Camp developed Montessori-based activities as a rehabilitation approach to the treatment of dementia (Orsulic-Jeras, Judge, & Camp, 2000).

In 1994, Dr. Bill Thomas publicly declared what we all knew, that nursing facilities were filled with residents who felt lonely, helpless, and bored; this statement has helped to humanize nursing facilities. His Eden Alternative philosophy has developed into an "international not-for-profit organization dedicated to transforming care environments into habitats for human beings that promote quality of life for all involved" (www.edenalt.org). The Eden Alternative (Thomas, 2004) is now being taught to care partners outside the long-term care setting in a program called Eden at Home, which is designed to touch the lives of older adults living at home as well as their care partners. Dr. Bill Thomas has also created "the Green House project, a radically new approach to long term care where nursing homes are torn down and replaced with small, home-like environments where people can live a full and interactive life" (changingaging.org/the-green-house-project).

Betsy Brawley (1997), an interior designer whose mother had Alzheimer's disease, wrote about creating dementia environments that support life. Margaret P. Calkins, an internationally recognized leader in the field of environments for elderly, especially those with Alzheimer's and other dementias, founded I.D.E.A.S., Inc. (Innovative Designs in Environments for an Aging Society), whose mission is "to engage in research, education, and consultation on the therapeutic potential of the environment—organizational and social as well as physical—particularly as it relates to frail and impaired older adults ... particularly those with Alzheimer's disease and other dementias" (www.ideasconsultinginc.com/Default.asp). All these innovators have increased health care professionals' and family care partners' knowledge about how to help people with Alzheimer's live with their disease.

## CULTURE CHANGE

The Pioneer Network gave birth to the notion of culture change that is sweeping the United States. This movement began in 1997 when a group of pioneering resident advocates and health care professionals agreed it was time to join forces to transform nursing facilities into places offering person-directed care that restored control to elders and their caregivers (www.pioneernetwork.net). The concept of culture change has come to mean a transformational change in a facility's values, practices, and day-to-day care culture. It has translated into changes in many of the nursing facilities in which I work, with positive results for both residents and staff. The following examples of culture change have helped remind the facility's staff members why they chose to work in a nursing facility.

## EPOCH SENIOR HEALTHCARE

> To get department managers out of their offices and away from their paperwork, EPOCH Senior Healthcare of Harwich, Massachusetts, decided that everyone had to lead at least one resident activity each month. The director of nursing played the piano and led a sing-along. The administrator met with residents to discuss her favorite subject, cooking. They chose a recipe from the administrator's cookbooks and then prepared the dish. The maintenance director led a men's group called Guess What This Is? in which he showed a tool and had the men guess how it is used. The staff and residents came to know each other better by getting together outside their usual roles and in a more casual setting.

Another EPOCH Senior Healthcare facility located in Brewster, Massachusetts, transformed one of its traditional 30-year-old units into a neighborhood by removing most of one nursing station and wallpapering the wall to look like a park. The remainder of the nursing station is hidden behind lattice work so that the nurses can still see the corridor. The bathroom was made to look more home-like, with colorful shower curtains and pictures of old-fashioned bathtubs. The day room was transformed into a country kitchen with brightly colored walls, a refrigerator, and a sink. Old wallpaper was torn down in the corridors, they were repainted a soft blue, and interesting and interactive art was hung on the walls; we replaced the "institutional" name plate on each door by installing a mailbox with the resident's name and the room number along with a sign welcoming visitors. This was a creative way to meet signage regulations and make this "mature" nursing facility look more like a place where people would want to live.

Another example of the philosophical changes occurring in nursing facilities in the United States is the Nursing Home Quality Initiative of the Centers for Medicare & Medicaid Services (CMS). This initiative promotes the transformation of nursing facilities from institutional to person-centered care models (CMS, 2012). Surveyors are no longer satisfied with seeing a room full of residents in an activity. Now they want to know whether residents had a choice in attending the program and whether they are engaged in the activity. A simple head count is not enough, especially if many participants are sleeping. They also want to know whether care partners really know the residents they are responsible for, who they are as unique individuals.

With no cure in sight and the average life expectancy increasing (age is the greatest risk factor for Alzheimer's disease), greater awareness of the need for specialized Alzheimer's services has emerged. Adult day service centers have become an option for families who choose to provide care at home and need respite during the day. Along with this service, home health companies are providing specialized services to families of clients with dementia as they meet the challenges of keeping their loved ones at home. The care of people with Alzheimer's disease is a thriving business, and with what we know now about how to provide thoughtful, affirming, high-quality care, we have begun the exciting process that will ultimately make nursing facilities and assisted living communities places where people, regardless of their physical or cognitive status, can live surrounded by caring team members.

## PEOPLE WITH ALZHEIMER'S DISEASE FIND THEIR VOICES

Since 1994, when Ronald Reagan wrote his poignant letter telling the American people that he had Alzheimer's disease, it has become easier for people with Alzheimer's disease and their families to talk about the experience of living with the disease. Families are writing books on various aspects of caring for someone with dementia. Newly diagnosed people are coming forward to speak about the disease; many are outspoken advocates for more research funds and better care. Richard Taylor (2007), a former psychologist who was diagnosed with early Alzheimer's disease, is a crusader for the newly diagnosed person with Alzheimer's disease. He established a large electronic network and e-mailed the following message on January 24, 2007:

> Stand up! So as not to become a victim of your own silence. Speak for yourself and those who will follow. Ask Carers and Friends to do the same. Today will never be here again. Time is of the Essence! Use it wisely!!! Tell as many people as possible your perceptions of your interactions with professionals, with carers, with friends, with strangers, with your government. They won't change unless they know, and they can't know unless and until you SPEAK UP! Seek to create a Palpable Sense of Change and of urgency! Join a Crusade, Now! Be a Crusader, Now! Lead a Crusade, Now!

Richard Taylor is one of many people with an irreversible dementia who are raising their voices to be heard at professional conferences and in the halls of Congress. They are demanding that money should be spent not only to find a cure for Alzheimer's disease but to find out how to help people with Alzheimer's disease live with quality in their lives and to give people with Alzheimer's disease a voice in policy decisions.

At a recent international conference I heard members of a group from Scotland called Scottish Dementia Working Group, which is run by people with dementia. They are "the independent voice of people with dementia within Alzheimer Scotland. The Working Group campaigns to improve services for people with dementia and to improve attitudes towards people with dementia" (www.sdwg.org.uk/). They have a voice in legislation regarding Alzheimer's disease, meet with ministers and other politicians, speak at conferences, and participate in the training of doctors, nurses, and social workers. This is just one of many advocacy organizations that are run by people with an irreversible dementia who are helping to raise issues that are important to people living with the disease.

## THE COST OF ALZHEIMER'S DISEASE

Billions of dollars are spent each year on research to find the cause and risk factors for Alzheimer's disease. However, a cure continues to be elusive. Medications are now available to slow the progression of the disease, but it has been many years since new ones have become available. We inch closer to finding the reasons why some people develop Alzheimer's disease and why others do not. When we know why, perhaps we can short-circuit the process and eliminate this disease. Until that day arrives, the number of people with dementia grows at an alarming rate; almost 50% of those older than 85 years of age develop Alzheimer's disease, and the number of people with early onset, before the age of 65, has reached 200,000 in the United States. Every 68 seconds another American develops Alzheimer's disease (Alzheimer's Association, 2012c). It appears that if we do not find a way to prevent or cure Alzheimer's disease, it may bankrupt our health care system; in fact, we may have already done so.

The toll on families is astronomical from both a financial and an emotional standpoint. In 2011, 15.2 million families and friends provided 17.4 billion hours of unpaid care for people with Alzheimer's disease and other dementias; about $210.5 billion is the estimated cost of this care (Alzheimer's Association, 2012c). The average cost of a room in a nursing facility is $85,775 for a private room and $75,555 for a semiprivate room. Assisted living communities charge a base rate of $55,428 a year on average (Met Life, 2011b), depleting family funds in many situations. Sadly, the toll on the family remains even after the death of their loved one, with one third reporting symptoms of depression (Alzheimer's Association, 2012c).

Prevention has become the new battle cry of the Alzheimer's Association. In response to aging baby boomers' fear of developing Alzheimer's disease, the association launched a campaign, Maintain Your Brain, with the message to "use your brain, exercise, and live a healthy lifestyle" (Alzheimer's Association, 2012a). How lovely it would be if my great-grandchildren could live without the fear of developing Alzheimer's disease. My dream is that one day hardly anyone will remember what Alzheimer's disease even was. Those of us who care for people with Alzheimer's disease would be gloriously out of work!

## CREATING NAMASTE CARE

Namaste Care™ was created in the spring of 2003, but the seeds had been planted years before. In 1981, while I was getting my master's degree in social work at the University of Minnesota and working part time in Westwood Nursing Home, I crossed paths with Robert Fulton, a sociology professor who had studied in London with Dame Cicely Sanders, the founder of the modern hospice movement. He offered a course on the hospice movement that introduced me to this special way of caring for people who are dying.

My first thoughts were that hospice was a great concept for residents in nursing facilities who were dying and in varying levels of pain or just seemed to be uncomfortable. Pain management was not as well understood as it is today. Pain medication was not administered until the resident complained. Then it took some time to take effect and was not administered again until the pain reappeared. This vicious cycle of pain kept many residents uncomfortable for many hours of the day and night. Nurses were also reluctant to give adequate doses of morphine because they feared it would hasten death or create an addiction.

In addition, to qualify for the Medicare hospice benefit, the patient had to have a "home" and "family caregiver." A nursing facility did not qualify on either count. Believing that there is more than one way to get around a regulation, I worked with the nursing facility staff to develop a hospice-like approach and do it ourselves.

With Professor Fulton's support and with guidance from the local hospice organization, we began our own end-of-life care. This would not have happened without the dynamic leadership of administrator Cheryl Nybo, fellow social worker Michael McDonough, and the great staff at Westwood Nursing Home. This incredible team believed that people should not die alone and in pain, so we changed the way our residents spent their last days. Hospice nurses helped with pain management according to what we knew about decreasing pain at that time, and we recruited alert, oriented residents to sit by the bedsides of dying residents, giving them comfort.

Sitting by the bedside of the dying was a time-honored tradition for the older generation and was not feared by them. One resident told me that in doing this service she finally felt worthwhile—that she still could do something that mattered. I'll never forget the look on one resident's face as she struggled into the room to take her turn at the bedside. She was as big as a minute and very frail. At my suggestion that maybe this was too much for her, she pulled herself up to her full four-foot-two height and declared that she was perfectly capable and I should mind my own business. I quickly backed out of the room. It would be very difficult to find nursing home residents who could do this now because most of them have dementia or are very physically debilitated.

It was not just other residents who sat with the dying. We enlisted everyone's help. Staff members were encouraged to do their paperwork and charting by the bedside of dying residents, just to be present for them. The dietary department made popsicles and lollipops for the residents to suck to help prevent the dry mouth that can be a problem at the end of life. The maintenance worker took his truck to a resident's house, packed up her china cabinet with figurines she had collected all her life, and reassembled it in her room so that she could spend her last days looking at her treasures. One resident wanted to attend religious services but was in too much pain to leave her bed, so staff members pushed her, bed and all, to the service. We were very creative in helping our residents live their last days peacefully, with someone sitting by their bedside whenever possible. In this second edition I have added information about the No One Dies Alone program, which I helped institute in a nursing facility (see Chapter 9).

When the Medicare Hospice Benefit was originally enacted, the typical patient had cancer and was verbal and could express feelings about dying. They could choose to receive hospice services. The patient with dementia was not even considered appropriate for receiving hospice services. That belief has changed. We now know that conversation at the end of life is not necessary and may not be desired; many patients just want to know that someone is there and that they are not alone.

Eventually, Medicare recognized nursing facility and assisted living residents as being eligible for the Medicare hospice benefit. However, few residents elected to use the benefit. Hospice workers were familiar only with patients who had cancer and were alert and oriented; they knew how to care for the residents physically and emotionally but were not comfortable caring for residents with dementia. My attempts to get my employers interested in encouraging hospice care in our communities were never very successful.

In 1994, I crossed paths with Ladislav Volicer, clinical director of the Geriatric Research, Education and Clinical Center at the Edith Nourse Rogers Memorial Veterans Hospital in Bedford, Massachusetts. Dr. Volicer was medical director of the Dementia Special Care Unit and pioneered the hospice approach to care for patients with late-stage dementia. His research has systematically evaluated the effects of palliative care options and led to the development of policies to guide hospice care that have affected U.S. public policy and the Medicare hospice benefit for people with advanced dementia. Dr. Volicer is a recognized expert in many medical aspects of palliative care.

Using the work of Dr. Volicer and his colleagues, we developed the Bethany Program for Hillhaven. Under the guidance of Nancy Orr-Rainey, we tried with limited success to interest our nursing facilities and the local hospice organization to form a partnership. We included residents with dementia among those we believed would qualify for the Medicare hospice benefit, but at that time, the number of residents with advanced dementia was low because this was not a diagnosis that was accepted under the hospice benefit. By 2010, the number of patients with a diagnosis of dementia had risen to 11.2% of hospice patients, and this figure does not take into consideration the number of patients listed under "debility" (13.1%), who often also have Alzheimer's disease. Unfortunately, it continues to be difficult to get anyone with dementia accepted into hospice care. The requirement for doctors to make a prognosis of "6 months to live" continues to limit referrals of dementia patients to hospice. Many physicians are not as enlightened as Dr. Volicer;

they believe that hospice care for someone with dementia is a waste of taxpayers' money. This is just another ongoing battle for people who have Alzheimer's disease. Hospice organizations, however, are now seeing the need to serve people with dementia and educate their staff about the unique needs of these patients.

In 2001, I began to consult with the Vermont Veterans Home, a nursing facility in Bennington, Vermont. My role as a consultant was to develop a unique program for residents on the secured dementia unit. The first program we developed was The Club, a program of continuous activities. The Club has shown that helping residents engage in meaningful activities throughout their waking hours made an impact in their lives and produced positive results (Simard & Volicer, 2002). The Club helped to decrease falls, the use of psychotropic medication, and social isolation. Residents gained weight, and staff and family satisfaction significantly increased. The Club also helped to fill empty beds. The unit filled quickly and began to boast a waiting list. However, even when residents were so advanced in their disease that they did not seem to benefit from the continuous programming, families did not want them to leave the unit. C Wing had become special not only because of its excellent care but also because of The Club. We needed to create another special program that would offer a different type of programming for residents who no longer could benefit from The Club and entice families to move their loved ones off C Wing when the time came.

The administrator at the Bennington facility, Earle Hollings, asked me to create a unique program for residents with advanced dementia. His vision was to expand the dementia program without simply re-creating another club. A wing on another unit became the location for a new program, Namaste. The programming we now call "meaningful activities" was based on some of the creative techniques that Mary Longtin, a restorative aide, had been using on C Wing for with residents with advanced dementia. With support of the administrator and all levels of staff, including director of nursing Marlene Restino, charge nurse Jennie LaBrake, dementia program director Christina Cosgrove, activity director Michele Burgess, and the staff of B Wing, we began creating the Namaste Care program.

With no budget, only an admonition to keep the costs as low as possible, we started Namaste Care in an activity room made to look less institutional with Goodwill furniture and donations of plants, quilts, and other old but interesting items. Thanks to the insight and talents of Mary Longtin, the first dedicated Namaste Carer, programming started with the basics of good nursing care. The residents' expressions told us that they enjoyed hand and foot massages. Other pleasurable activities included listening to music, inhaling the scent of lavender, and receiving gentle touches. The presence of others, especially the soft murmuring of voices, seemed to lower residents' anxiety. We realized that we could make a positive difference in the lives of residents who had shown little response to activities in The Club. Their families noticed a positive change in their loved ones and were delighted with the attention given to this new program. They told us that visiting time was easier when they sat in the Namaste Care room. Residents who had been crying out for help stopped this anxiety-related behavior, residents who had lost all verbal skills would spontaneously say something, and residents who had no or little reaction to stimuli smiled when bubbles were blown their way. Small miracles happened almost every day (Simard, 2012a). Everyone was happy: residents, families, staff, and surveyors. It was so simple: Create a calm, peaceful setting, slow everything down, always touch with love, treat everyone as a unique individual, respect choice, and, above all, honor the spirit within. It seems that we have a great deal to learn about living from our care of the dying.

## Teach Me to Die

Teach me to die
Hold on to my hand
I have so many questions
Things I don't understand
Teach me to die
Give me all you can give
If you'll teach me of dying
I will teach you to live
*Deanna Edwards*

Staff and family who were involved with this first Namaste Care program were so pleased that we realized it needed to be spread beyond the confines of this one facility. Christina Cosgrove, Michele Burgess, Dr. Volicer, and I began speaking about the program at conferences. Dr. Volicer and I presented the Namaste Care program on speaking engagements in Australia and Asia. People often remarked that no one else was offering this specialized care and asked where they could find more information about it. I was not comfortable with the idea of writing a book, but then my presence at the death of Matthew Wilk changed everything.

## MATTHEW'S STORY

Matthew was part of Namaste Care for several months before he died. I had seen the pleasure on his face when he was placed in a comfortable lounge chair and offered orange slices and lollipops. He was in the presence of other residents who were also in the last stages of dementia-related illnesses, not isolated in his room or asleep in The Club. He spent the majority of the day with caring Namaste Care team members, in a room filled with beautiful music and the scent of lavender drifting through the air. Namaste Care team members offered Matthew a variety of meaningful activities, such as receiving hand and foot massages, listening to the sounds of nature, and hearing gentle conversations. Matthew spent the last months of his life in this comforting place with his wife, Celia, often at his side.

Matthew Wilk died on July 12, 2004. Matthew was a husband to Celia for 56 years, a father of five, a retired transformer specialist for General Electric for 35 years, and a person who had lived with dementia for 6 years.

Because of his participation in the Namaste Care program, Matthew's last weeks could have been sad; they were not. Matthew's last days could have been heartbreaking; they were not. Matthew's last hours could have been distressing; they were not. Matthew's death could have been devastating; it was not. Matthew left this world with dignity, love, and compassionate care and on the wings of laughter (Simard, 2005).

Several months after Matthew's death, his wife, Celia, and I were sitting in the private room reserved for Namaste Care residents. This was the room where Matthew spent his last days, where he died. She looked around the room and gave a rueful smile at what had transpired in the room, the place where her wonderful husband died, recognizing what a beautiful passing it was. We realized that the passing of Matthew had made a difference in both our lives. For Celia, it was the end of a journey for her husband, who had struggled with dementia for so many years. For me, it was being present during his death and seeing how the Namaste Care program had taken on a life of its own and blossomed in ways I never anticipated. Namaste Care could really make a difference in the way people with advanced dementia lived their last days and how they died. I needed to tell its story. Just as storytellers have taught lessons of life for thousands of years, Namaste Care will be illustrated through this book as the story of Matthew Wilk—one of his final gifts.

# CHAPTER 2

# What Is Namaste Care?

*Namaste*
I honor the place in you in which the entire Universe
dwells, I honor the place in you which is of Love, of
Truth, of Light and of Peace. When you are in that
place in you, and I am in that place in me, we are One.

The word *Namaste*, pronounced "nah-ma-stā," is a Hindu greeting most often heard in the United States from yoga instructors
as a farewell to students at the end of class. Two hands are pressed
together and held near the heart with the head gently bowed as the
person says, "Namaste. Go in peace." The word *Namaste* expresses
a wish to honor the spirit within and was selected as the name to describe a special way of caring for residents in a nursing facility or an
assisted living community as well as hospice patients with advanced
dementia or another life-limiting illness.

## THE PHILOSOPHY AND MISSION STATEMENT

The foundation of any program is an idea, a philosophy. The Namaste Care™ philosophy supports the belief that the spirit of residents with advanced dementia continues to live. We see the spirit
in residents' eyes, their smiles, and their response to a loving touch.
This is this spirit that is undaunted by disease, the spirit beyond the
disease. It is the essence of a person.

Namaste Care Philosophy Statement

We believe that the spirit in each person lives regardless of their physical and cognitive status and that it is possible to nurture this spirit in each individual through loving touch and meaningful activities. This spirit thrives when residents are in the presence of others.

Whereas a philosophy is what you believe, the mission statement is what you do.

Namaste Care Mission Statement

Namaste Care is provided by an interdisciplinary team of compassionate and knowledgeable health care professionals as well as families and friends. A holistic approach to care ensures that the burdens and benefits of each medical intervention or nursing treatment are weighed so that they support each person's quality of life. Comfort and pleasure are the goals of Namaste Care. Every effort is made so that quality-of-life experiences are offered every day throughout a person's time in Namaste Care. The team will also do everything possible in the person's final stage of life so that the dying process is a pain-free, easy passing surrounded by people who care.

This is a sample mission statement, but I urge each organization offering Namaste Care to create their own. It can be a statement written by Namaste Carers assigned to the program. The two Namaste Carers at EPOCH Senior Healthcare of Brewster, Massachusetts, Barbara Holmes and Janet Gilmour, wrote a mission statement for their Namaste Care program. It hangs on the wall as you enter the Namaste Care room. It is simple yet eloquent.

Namaste Care Mission

To embrace our most vulnerable and provide them with a sense of comfort, calmness and serenity because their lives are still relevant

Love Is Our Religion

If the Namaste Care room is located in a neighborhood, all team members should be involved in writing the mission statement, with someone designated as a facilitator. When I am the facilitator, I schedule team members' meetings for each shift and include care partners, housekeeping, maintenance, dietary, activities, and any auxiliary team members usually assigned to the neighborhood. It is more effective to hold these meetings after Namaste Care has been in place for a few weeks so that team members can actually see it and experience the changes they observe in residents. At the meetings, I use a flip chart to write what they say about the program and their goals for residents in Namaste Care. I try to capture not only the words and sentences team members suggest but how they personally feel about Namaste Care. I periodically review with them what I have written to make sure I have captured their thoughts correctly. After I have reached as many team members as possible, I write a draft of their mission statement, using as many of their words as possible. The draft mission statement is then passed out to all team members. They are asked for feedback, and any changes or additions are made. When the mission statement has been approved by the majority of the team, it is presented to the administrator or person in charge for approval.

The final mission statement is printed on high-quality paper and framed with a wide mat. Each team member working on the neighborhood or assigned to Namaste Care signs the matting. The framed mission statement is hung on the wall of the Namaste Care room and serves as a reminder to everyone that they are entering a special place. Copies are given to orient all new team members assigned to the neighborhood or to the Namaste Care program and after the 90-day probation period, they are asked to sign the matting as a symbol of their commitment to Namaste Care.

## THE NAMASTE CARE PROGRAM OVERVIEW

Namaste Care is a 7-day-a-week program because Alzheimer's disease is a 7-day-a-week disease. It is sensory based and is led and supervised primarily by nursing, although all team members, including management, have some responsibilities to ensure that it takes place every day for at least 4 hours a day. Activities of daily living (ADLs) are offered with a loving approach and are the meaningful activities that make up the substance of the Namaste Care day.

The Namaste Care program takes place in a designated room as free as possible from distractions and noise. If space is limited, it can be located in a dual-purpose room that, for instance, may also be used for dining or activities. In preparation for the Namaste Care program, carers create a tranquil, serene environment in the space by lowering the lights and eliminating distractions such as overhead paging and call lights. Soothing music is played, the scent of lavender permeates the room, and the décor is warm and inviting. If the space is used for other purposes, items such as tablecloths and flowers may be used to "stage" it during the Namaste Care program. Supplies are gathered before the room is opened so that residents are never left alone.

Each resident is greeted and welcomed to Namaste Care. All team members are responsible for transporting residents to the Namaste Care room. They are also asked to help the person designated to lead the program, referred to as the Namaste Carer, transfer residents from wheelchairs to comfortable lounge chairs if their wheelchairs cannot be adjusted for maximum relaxation. Residents are assessed for pain or discomfort (see Appendix F), and quilts or soft blankets are tucked around them so that they feel warm and secure. Uncomfortable shoes may be replaced with warm soft socks, belts may be removed or loosened, and pillows are used for positioning.

The Namaste Carer will have received special education regarding advanced dementia. He or she will also have been shown how to provide a variety of meaningful activities throughout the Namaste Care day. In the morning, activities include gently washing the resident's face, hands, and arms, then applying moisturizing lotion and tenderly brushing their hair. Each resident is offered beverages throughout the day because people with advanced dementia are often malnourished. Beverages include a variety of juices, water, or shakes. Residents who are not in danger of choking may also enjoy lollipops, fresh orange or banana slices, ice cream, and puddings. A list of residents attending Namaste Care who have diet restrictions or need liquids thickened is always kept current and available to the Namaste Carer.

Before lunch, the Namaste Carer changes the feeling in the room to provide more stimulation so residents are awake and more alert for lunch. Lights are turned up, and livelier music is played. Fun sensory objects such as realistic-looking birds that chirp, wind chimes, puppets, and seasonal or holiday items are shown to residents. Namaste Carers also use natural items to offer an awareness of the season to each resident. They may use freshly cut grass in a basket during the summer, seasonal fresh flowers almost year round, and colorful and interesting-looking gourds in the fall. One wintery New England day, a creative Namaste Carer asked me to stay with the residents while she left the room. She returned with several basins of snow that she placed on the residents' laps I'll never forget the expressions of glee on the residents' faces as they tried to make snowballs! Even in the advanced stage of dementia, residents can continue to have fun,

The room closes about 15 or 20 minutes before lunch. The assigned care partners take the residents to their rooms to be changed. As they leave the Namaste Care room, residents are thanked for attending and invited back for the afternoon program. After lunch some residents are taken to their rooms for a nap, and others return for the afternoon session. Residents may attend Namaste Care for the entire day or part of the day, depending on their physical status.

Family members and friends are encouraged to visit the Namaste Care room and become part of the program by giving their loved ones a hand massage, brushing their hair, or helping them eat ice cream or drink juice. Some families just enjoy holding hands with their loved ones and talking to other family members in the room, especially when their family member is nonverbal. Namaste Carers often report that family visits are longer and that some families volunteer to spend time with residents who do not have visitors. Occasionally families will take their loved ones out of the room for a stroll in the courtyard or they visit in the residents' rooms for some private time. Families and team members are encouraged to come into the Namaste Care room anytime they wish. Medications may be dispensed to residents in the room if it can be done without wheeling the medication cart into the room. Medical procedures are to be provided in the privacy of a resident's room.

Residents are welcomed to Namaste Care as they enter the room for the afternoon session. Residents who did not attend the morning program have their faces and hands washed and moisturized and their hair brushed. Those who did attend the morning program are offered activities that were different from what they received earlier in the day. They may have their feet soaked and lotion applied to their feet and legs. Some residents enjoy range-of-motion exercises to dance music. This brings pleasure to the residents and helps keep their limbs flexible. A nature video may be playing for residents who are awake, and shoulder rubs are offered while they watch the video. Before the room closes for the day, lights are again turned up and music such as sing-alongs or show tunes are played and a variety of food scents may be available to stimulate the residents' appetite for dinner. Each resident is thanked for attending Namaste Care and hugged good-bye. The Namaste Carer completes paperwork and tidies the room for the next day. More information is available on the Namaste Care day in Chapter 5.

## NAMASTE CARE OUTCOMES

Since the inception of Namaste Care, I have been involved in a few research projects looking at outcomes. One showed a decrease in the need for antianxiety medications (Simard & Volicer, 2010). Another pilot study for the School of Nursing, University of Western Sydney, Australia, found that staff and family satisfaction were greater in a high-touch model of care than in a high-tech model. Most of the outcomes are anecdotal evidence from nursing staff, carers, and families, who report positive changes in behavior that resulted in lowering of the use of antipsychotic medication. I hear from nurses and carers that team members are happier with their work when Namaste Care is offered to people with advanced dementia. I have rarely heard of a Namaste Care program stopping once it began.

## NAMASTE CARE STANDARDS

To maintain the integrity of Namaste Care, the program must have standards. I have tried to make those standards flexible enough to apply to health care providers in skilled nursing facilities and assisted living communities. Each standard can be met in a variety of ways that give the program credibility. Additional information has been written on each standard in other chapters. The standards for Namaste Care are as follows.

### Namaste Care Is Offered 7 Days a Week

Alzheimer's disease and other end-of-life diseases and conditions never take a day off, and neither should Namaste Care. Residents in the program need and deserve high-quality programming 7 days a week. I do recognize that long-term care is a very human business, with sick days, vacation days, and the dreaded "call outs" that occur, making staffing 7 days a week challenging. When there is a dedicated Namaste Carer in addition to regular care staff, filling in for emergencies is not difficult. However, as states and the federal government continue to cut reimbursement, adding staff is a cost many facilities cannot justify.

Flexibility is the key to meeting this standard. Supported by the culture-change movement, lines between management and team members' job responsibilities should be less rigid. After all, it is everyone's responsibility to care for and about our residents, and training every team member to work in Namaste Care will help ensure that Namaste Care is offered 7 days a week. If the team member is not a qualified or certified nursing assistant or nurse, he or she can still comb residents' hair, moisturize their hands, or read to them. The most important service they can offer is their presence in the room. Chapter 3 provides additional information on staffing the Namaste Care daily program.

### Namaste Care Is Offered at Least 4 Hours a Day

Namaste Care is offered in the morning and afternoon. Residents in Namaste Care spend many hours in bed, so the 4 hours in the Namaste Care room, with meals in the dining room, decreases their isolation and is an important element of their quality of life. The typical Namaste Care day is explained in Chapter 5.

### Namaste Care Takes Place in a Special Environment

Namaste Care is located in a space or room whose environmental features support the loving approach to providing meaningful activities. This includes soft lighting, calming music, and the scent of lavender or another appropriate scent. The room is made to look as home-like and inviting as possible. The Namaste Care setting is detailed in Chapter 4.

### Residents Are Assessed for Comfort

Quality of life is not possible if a resident is not comfortable and pain free. Each resident is assessed for comfort as part of his or her participation in Namaste Care, using a variety of assessment tools and the judgment of the Namaste Carer. A means of communicating to nursing staff any concern about pain and discomfort must be established in each facility.

### Residents Who Receive Psychoactive Medications Are Assessed by Nursing Staff for Changes in Behavior

Residents' behavior treated with psychoactive medications sometimes change when they become involved in Namaste Care. It is not surprising if they change the day they begin attending Namaste Care. The nursing department must develop a way to assess residents who attend Namaste Care and who are receiving psychoactive medications at least bi-monthly. Someone on the nursing staff must also come to the Namaste Care program at least once a day to assess residents' comfort and note changes in behavior. In the past, medications were not reviewed until it was time for a care plan or wellness plan review, leaving residents on medications that were no longer necessary. The government has set goals for discontinuing antipsychotic medications, and the Namaste Care program can help meet those goals.

### Activities of Daily Living Are Offered as Meaningful Activities

ADLs and other activities are offered throughout the morning and afternoon sessions. They include washing the resident's face and hands, applying moisturizer, and gently combing their hair. Sensory items used to increase awareness of the seasons and holidays must be kept current. Chapter 5 outlines a variety of meaningful activities.

### After-Death Care Ritual

When a resident dies the body is prepared for the funeral home. At least one team member accompanies the resident out of the facility to the hearse as a special way of honoring him or her even after death. The after-death ritual is explained in Chapter 9.

### After-Death Evaluation

Within 7 days of a resident's death, a meeting is scheduled with team members to discuss whether anyone thinks any improvement could have been made in the resident's care. The meeting ends with a review of what they did to make this death a peaceful transition for the resident and his or her family.

## CRITERIA AND A PROCESS FOR DETERMINING WHICH RESIDENTS ARE APPROPRIATE FOR RECEIVING NAMASTE CARE

In order to determine who will be served by Namaste Care, admissions or participation guidelines need to be developed and written. These guidelines help team members, families, other professionals, and state surveyors understand the physical and cognitive status of the population to be served. Most residents in Namaste Care will have a diagnosis of an advanced irreversible dementia or similar symptoms, as well as the following:

- Inability to actively participate in activity programs

- Difficulty communicating

- Need for assistance with most personal care

- Inability to ambulate

- Receiving psychoactive medications

The most import qualification is that team members feel as if Namaste Care will improve the resident's quality of life.

## Alzheimer's Disease

The following overview of Alzheimer's disease is taken from the Alzheimer's Association web site (www.alz.org/index.asp). This is an excellent resource that is constantly updated.

People with Alzheimer's disease are the primary participants in Namaste Care programs. Alzheimer's disease is a progressive, irreversible brain disorder that gradually destroys a person's memory and ability to learn, reason, make judgments, communicate, and carry out daily activities. People with Alzheimer's disease may also experience changes in their personalities and may have hallucinations or delusions. At this time no cure for Alzheimer's disease is available and no drugs significantly slow its progression.

It is believed that Alzheimer's disease is caused by a number of factors, including genetic predisposition. Some families have a history of early-onset Alzheimer's disease, and other people have genes known to increase the risk of developing Alzheimer's disease. It is well known that age is the greatest risk factor for developing Alzheimer's disease; the probability of having Alzheimer's disease is almost 50% by age 85.

Environmental factors such as stress, head injury, and low education are also high on the list of risk factors for developing Alzheimer's disease. Research indicates that if a person is intellectually stimulated, exercises regularly, controls his or her blood pressure, and maintains low cholesterol levels, he or she lowers the chances of developing Alzheimer's disease.

The first signs of Alzheimer's disease are usually significant short-term memory loss, increased confusion, and difficulty with shopping and household tasks. A visit to a physician is necessary to rule out any reversible causes for these symptoms. As part of the diagnostic work-up, physicians will take a physical history, give the person a thorough medical exam, run laboratory tests, and conduct various neurological and memory tests. Ultimately, a diagnosis of Alzheimer's disease is not certain until death, when an autopsy can confirm the presence of amyloid plaques and neurofibrillary tangles in the brain.

The diagnosis of Alzheimer's disease may be complicated because of the presence of other related dementias, including vascular dementia, frontotemporal dementia, dementia with Lewy bodies, and Parkinson's disease. Although early-stage symptoms of these other dementias differ, by the advanced stage symptoms become very similar.

When a person is diagnosed with probable or possible Alzheimer's disease, one of the several medications that show promise in slowing the progression of the disease may be prescribed. The usual life span of a person with Alzheimer's disease is 8 years, although some live as long as 20 years with the disease.

Namaste Care has been designed for residents in the advanced stage of Alzheimer's disease or a related dementia. Residents in the advanced stage of their disease are usually unable to take part in typical daily activities and will benefit from the special programming provided as part of Namaste Care.

## Other Diagnoses or Conditions Suitable for Namaste Care

I mentioned that originally Namaste Care was developed for skilled nursing facilities and that it bloomed into a program for a variety of health care organizations. Another "bloom" occurred in my own perception of who would benefit from the program. Originally I believed it was for nursing home residents with advanced dementia and other end-of-life diseases and conditions. As I discovered, and continue to learn, residents with a variety of physical and cognitive problems benefit from the Namaste Care approach. Consider the story of Martha, a resident whose life was profoundly changed by Namaste Care.

### MARTHA

Martha, a resident in a nursing facility, had a diagnosis of mental illness. She had been a resident for 6 years and was quite alone. She was never married, and her closest relative was a nephew who visited infrequently. Martha was one of those residents who sits in front of the nurse's station and screams, "Help me!" Every facility has residents like Martha, and the team members are challenged and frustrated by them. No matter what they try to help soothe and calm, nothing seems to work. Martha cried out for help and complained of a headache. No amount of medication seemed to help her. No amount of handholding seemed to help her. She had every imaginable test over the years, and no clinical reason for her expression of pain could be found. Very few of the nursing and activity team members were able to connect with her in a meaningful way. Sometimes they could comfort her by placing a cool washcloth over her forehead; when care partners had the time, they sat by her side. Martha did not like to be touched, so giving personal care was a challenge. In desperation, team members brought her to the Namaste Care room. She was lifted from her wheelchair and placed in a comfortable lounge chair. A comforter was tucked under her chin. Then the miracle began.

Martha stopped screaming. The headache complaints ceased. She looked around the room and seemed pleased by what she saw. She still did not like to be touched by most team members, but she developed a very special relationship with a male care partner whom she allowed to care for her. When Martha hugged him, a beautiful expression appeared on her face; it was as if she finally had a son. Martha enjoyed sucking on lollipops and watching nature videos from her favorite chair. She seemed to appreciate the quiet environment of the room, and although she did not actively engage in activities, she showed that she was aware of her surroundings. The "new Martha" was easier for team members to approach. On the day she died, a year later, a Namaste Carer came in on her day off to hold Martha's hand. Clearly, Martha's happiest days of the last year of her life were spent in Namaste Care.

## Another small miracle occurred with Evelyn (Simard, 2012a).

### EVELYN

Evelyn was haunted by hallucinations of her past, when she was a police dispatcher. She was reliving the frantic calls from people in a crisis. Evelyn constantly murmured into her clenched fist as if it were a microphone, "They are dying, look at all the blood, oh, the children, the poor children." This and other cries for help had her trapped in an ongoing nightmare. Staff had found no way of calming her, and although a variety of medications had been prescribed, none were successful in wiping these horrible visions from her memory. It took several days in the Namaste Care room and the compassionate care offered by Namaste Carer Chris Donovan, but eventually Evelyn was freed her from her world of pain and suffering. The hallucinations gradually drifted away, and she was actually a happy person who smiled and loved Chris. One day when I was visiting the program, she asked Chris to get her a teapot and stated that she would pay her 12 cents for it. I stayed with the residents while Chris went to the dining room and got a teapot. For the next 30 minutes, Evelyn caressed the teapot and told stories of having friends over for tea, a miracle taking place right before our eyes. For the rest of her life, Evelyn was happy and comfortable (Simard, 2012a).

Like Martha and Evelyn, who didn't fit the usual profile for Namaste Care, another resident named Carl was frustrating to care for. Despite the many different approaches used with him, he seemed to be distressed and anxious most of the time.

## CARL

Carl was admitted to the dementia unit several years before the Namaste Care program. When first admitted to the facility, he was able to walk and occasionally joined activities. As the disease progressed, he gradually began to have problems with falling and was deemed unsafe to walk on his own. He was evaluated by a physical therapist and, after breaking several wheelchairs, was given a special rocking wheelchair because he seemed to need to be constantly moving. Carl found a place in the corridor where he moved up and down throughout the day. He was resistive to care and from his expression seemed to be a very unhappy man.

The activity team members were unable to find anything that he enjoyed. Out of desperation, he was taken to the Namaste Care room, where he was placed in a lounge chair near the window. He seemed to be able to feel the sunlight, and he responded to this peaceful setting by falling asleep. When agitated, he was spoken to in a soft voice; he liked hearing about activities he had enjoyed in the past. One day when he became increasingly agitated, Mary Longtin, the Namaste Carer, knelt next to him and talked to him about his love of picking apples. His family had mentioned that this was one of his favorite activities each fall, and she used this as a way to honor his past. She gave him an item that provided the scent of apples and showed him pictures of apples. With a soft, soothing voice, she talked him through the ritual of apple picking; before long, Carl was asleep.

Nan was another surprise beneficiary of Namaste Care. All nursing facilities have residents who pace, and Nan was one of them. Team members find it difficult or impossible to get these residents to rest. There is a difference between pacing and wandering. The resident who is wandering can usually be redirected and engaged by team members. The resident who paces believes she has places to go and things to do and is not easily redirected.

*NAN*

Nan was a younger resident who had lived in the dementia neighborhood for several years. She had the most beautiful eyes and a smile that melted hearts, but she paced constantly. One day Nan found her way to the Namaste Care room. Perhaps it was the low lighting, the scent of lavender, the soft, soothing music, and the quiet atmosphere that called to her. Whenever she walked into the room, she headed for an empty chair, and for a few minutes she looked around the room before closing her eyes and going to sleep for 10 to 15 minutes. When she woke up, the Namaste Carer offered her something to drink and some ice cream. Because of her constant pacing, she was at high risk for weight loss, so any calories they could get her to consume were beneficial. So, for brief periods during the day, Nan appeared to welcome the peace of the Namaste Care room and was at rest.

Over the years, the variety of residents who can benefit from Namaste Care has reminded me never to give up on the quest for quality of life for anyone in our care. The person who taught me this valuable lesson was the late Barbara Holmes, who was a certified nursing assistant at EPOCH Senior Healthcare of Brewster, Massachusetts, for 25 years and one of the best Namaste Carers I ever worked with. Barbara rarely gave up on a resident. She would try to soothe someone who was crying out even if they could stay in the room for only 5 minutes. Perhaps by the next week they could stay for 10 minutes. Barbara always reminded me that even

10 minutes of peace and comfort was important to someone who was obviously in distress.

## ETHEL

> Ethel was another resident who paced constantly, seemingly looking for something but unable to communicate what that something was. Her face was pinched with concentration, and she rarely smiled. She was at risk for falling and weight loss, but it was impossible to have someone always at her side. Somehow, somewhere, Barbara found an enormous white stuffed dog and invited Ethel into the Namaste Room, where she seated her in a comfortable lounge chair that reclined, making it a bit more difficult for her to get up. Then, Barbara introduced this huge dog to her. Right before my eyes, a transformation took place; Ethel's sad face disappeared, replaced by a smile almost as huge as the dog. Barbara sat the dog on Ethel's lap and asked her to help care for it. The dog was so large, Ethel was overwhelmed with the sheer size of it, and rather than sending it flying across the room, as she did with a smaller version, she spent 30 minutes cuddling it and talking to it. Then another miracle occurred: This resident, who constantly paced, fell asleep holding the dog in her lap.

The lesson in these cases is that if team members, not just the nursing or activity staff, believe that the life of any resident could be improved by Namaste Care, go for it! And do not give up! Martha did not immediately stop crying out, nor did Evelyn stop having her disturbing hallucinations, but each day they could stay a bit longer until eventually they both spent the majority of each day peacefully and occasionally joyfully in the Namaste Care room.

Because the type of resident who will benefit from Namaste Care has changed so dramatically since the first edition of this book, I decided not to establish strict criteria for participation in the program. What I do want to see is that on a weekly or at least biweekly basis, team members are asked to update the list of participants. When a death occurs, another resident can quickly take the person's place in the Namaste Care room.

As promised, the story of a resident named Matthew Wilk embodies the essence of Namaste Care. He was one of the first participants in the program. His story begins with how he was selected for the program (Simard, 2005).

## MATTHEW'S STORY

Matthew was one of the first residents to participate in Namaste Care. He met the criteria for the program because he was no longer able to participate in activity programs, was not ambulatory, and needed total care. At first he could still respond to yes-and-no questions and motion to pictures placed in front of him. Gradually he lost all verbal communication and could communicate only with his eyes. Matthew seemed to recognize his wife, Celia, who visited often. Like so many spouses, Celia had tried valiantly to care for Matthew at home, at first on her own and then with adult day services. They had a wonderful marriage, as anyone could see from the light in Celia's eyes when she recalled their life together. Now, during the final months, it was increasingly difficult for Celia to visit. Matthew was slipping away, sleeping more than he was awake; it was difficult for him to respond to her words. Because he slept through the activity program on the dementia neighborhood, he was taken to the Namaste Care room for the special individualized sensory programs. Celia enjoyed giving her husband hand massages and visiting with the Namaste Carers and other spouses visiting their loved ones. Namaste Care provided both Matthew and Celia with a support group of caring people.

Matthew perfectly fit the criteria for Namaste Care. He received personalized care that identified him as a unique individual, and his personhood was not diminished in spite of the many losses he experienced because of his disease. His story shows how the philosophy and mission of Namaste Care can help those who are living with dementia maintain a life with moments of quality.

# CHAPTER 3

# The Namaste Care Team

The only way to do great work is to love what you do. If you haven't found it yet, keep looking. Don't settle. As with all matters of the heart, you'll know when you find it.

STEVE JOBS

This chapter will address what appears to be the major barrier that prevents a nursing facility or assisted living community from starting a Namaste Care™ program: the incorrect belief that additional team members, especially care partners, must be hired. Most people who hear about the Namaste Care program love the concept but think they do not have the resources to hire additional team members. Furthermore, management often justifies not offering Namaste Care because they think that care partners already provide most of what is offered in the program. However, if I ask, "Do you believe that care partners have time to give hand massages every day? Are your residents with advanced dementia offered programs of "meaningful activities" for at least 4 hours a day every day?" The answer is usually "No." In a good facility, care partners try to give hand or neck massages when they have time; they sit and talk with the residents when they have time. The problem is that they rarely have time. Activity professionals offer individual visits to residents who cannot participate in programming, but this usually occurs about three times a week and may last for less than 30 minutes, far less time than the daily programming in the Namaste Care room. Namaste Care strongly supports the belief that quality of life is more than keeping someone dressed, changed, groomed, and fed. Quality of life also includes the meaningful activities provided at least 4 hours a day 7 days a week in Namaste Care. When I see the anxious expressions or the flat affect on residents' faces disappear when bubbles are blown toward them and they playfully bat them away, or residents who usually do not speak spontaneously tell a care partner "I love you" while their hair is being brushed with slow loving strokes, I know that Namaste Care helps people with advanced dementia live a life with many moments of quality.

Namaste Care is not about having money for additional team members, expensive supplies, and equipment or having a dedicated room. It is about recognizing the psychosocial needs of residents, especially for those with advanced dementia, and having the heart to offer this end-of-life program. The only other requirement is that the facility team members work as a team. The success of implementing the program depends on everyone on the team, from management to team members, understanding that Namaste Care is everyone's responsibility. A true team effort will make the program happen 7 days a week. As Jason Chellun, proprietor of Lakeside Nursing Home in Upper Norwood in London, tells his team members: "Namaste is like lunch: it happens every day."

Creating an excellent Namaste Care program is all about hiring excellent team members. And excellent team members know their job and love what they do. The team is composed of management, nurses, care partners, activity professionals, housekeeping, maintenance, food service, and office staff; if you work in the facility, you are considered part of the team.

Based on 10 years of seeing programs and hearing from others how Namaste Care is implemented throughout the United States and in other countries, I will offer you examples of how to implement the program as part of an existing special dementia neighborhood, in a room that can be located anywhere in the facility, or in a Namaste Care neighborhood where the majority of residents are in the advanced stage of the disease.

## STAFFING A DEMENTIA SPECIAL CARE NEIGHBORHOOD

Many of the Namaste Care daily programs are part of a dementia special care neighborhood sometimes referred to as "memory care," where residents are in all stages of an irreversible dementia. The Namaste Care daily program may take place in a dedicated room or a dual-purpose space that is also the dining room or a family room. (More information on space options can be found in Chapter 4.) The morning Namaste Care program starts after breakfast and continues until about 30 minutes before lunch. The afternoon program begins after lunch and when the residents have been groomed and changed or toileted. It closes before dinner.

I think the most successful programs have two or three care partners designated as Namaste Carers who enjoy providing meaningful activities and are assigned to the Namaste Care room on a regular basis, one at a time. With at least three Namaste Carers, coverage can be provided 7 days a week and allow for vacations and illnesses. Designating three main Namaste Carers results in better communication between them about the likes and dislikes of individual residents, and they can get to know the families better. It is surprising to me that so many families whose loved one had been part of Namaste Care and had died continue to come to the Namaste Care room as volunteers, in part because they miss seeing the Namaste Carers who had become their extended family. I have also found that when the Namaste Carers feel ownership of their program, they make sure supplies are stocked and the room is clean and orderly. These dedicated Namaste Carers also reap the accolades from families and visitors. When I am introduced to the Namaste Carer and they tell me about their program, I see them light up with pride.

EPOCH Senior Living, a Massachusetts-based health care company, made the decision to hire Namaste Carers for their skilled facilities. Their family and staff satisfaction with Namaste Care is exceptional, and 8 years later, even with the financial cuts from Medicare and Medicaid, they have not cut these positions.

In the Arden Courts assisted living model, care partners have requested 30-minute rotations because they all want to be a part of the Namaste Care program. (More information on this assisted living experience can be found in Chapter 7.)

If there is not a dedicated Namaste Carer position, the responsibility for the daily program will be assigned to a care partner who also has an assignment of residents. In some facilities, the care partner who is responsible for Namaste Care may have a fewer number of assigned residents. The care partner who has been designated responsible for the daily program will see that notation (N) on his or her assignment list. In other cases, at the brief meeting with the charge nurse at the beginning of a new shift the nurse might ask who would like to do the daily program so that everyone on the team has an opportunity to be the Namaste Carer for the day or for a half day. When the team makes the decision, the quality of the program improves because it is not just an assignment; it is the care partner's choice. Care partners then begin their day by providing morning care and serving breakfast to the residents assigned to them. The care partner assigned to the Namaste Care room may not have all of his or her residents in the Namaste Care room. This is when the team concept is important. While the Namaste Carers have other care partners' residents in the room, some of the residents assigned to them may not be present, and are perhaps attending other activity programs. Others on the team are watching them. The number of residents in the Namaste Care room should be at least the number of residents in one care partner's assignment; therefore, the Namaste Carer is in fact taking one assignment.

We have been happily surprised to find that volunteers can be recruited for Namaste Care from church groups and senior citizen programs. Some hospice programs are training their volunteers to help add an extra pair of hands for the daily program. Every once in a while, I have heard that some alert residents have volunteered as Namaste volunteers. Their service helps to make them feel that even though they live in a nursing facility they can still help others.

In situations where Namaste Care is part of a larger community, such as one that offers independent living or traditional assisted living, volunteers can be recruited for Namaste Care. All volunteers, resident volunteers, and family members must be approved by the team member responsible for the volunteer program and receive orientation and may be required to have a background check and tuberculosis skin test before qualifying to volunteer.

Volunteers are never left alone in the Namaste Care room without a care partner present.

Activity professionals provide individual visits to residents who do not attend programming. If a number of these residents are in Namaste Care, some hours from that department can be scheduled in the Namaste Care room. An activity program for residents in the moderate stage of dementia should take place concurrently so that the few remaining residents who are not involved in either program can be looked after by any care partner on the team.

The calmness that becomes the norm in a special dementia neighborhood when the majority of the residents are busy is at first unbelievable to team members who are used to a sometimes chaotic atmosphere, and then a calm neighborhood becomes the norm. One of the best compliments I have heard was from a man fixing the security system in an elevator for a third-floor dementia special care neighborhood. This facility offered The Club for residents with moderate dementia and Namaste Care for residents with advanced dementia. The neighborhood was quiet except for a few residents quietly wandering in the corridors and a few residents who chose not to participate in either program. This technician told the maintenance manager, "I thought you said this was a dementia floor?" He worked with security for dementia programs every day and had never experienced the quiet and peace of this neighborhood.

## TEAM EDUCATION

As with any new program, education is the first step. The entire special care team attends in-services about Namaste Care programming, and everyone is encouraged to ask questions about it. All care partners are told that if they are interested in being selected to work in the Namaste Care room as a Namaste Carer, they should let the neighborhood manager know. Not all care partners are creative, and providing meaningful activities might not be something they would enjoy. The meaningful activities offered in Namaste Care are focused on process, not task, and not all care partners are suited to this slow approach to care. However, beware of making assumptions about which team members are best suited to the program and which would not. Sometimes the most task-oriented care partner, someone you would never expect to enjoy Namaste Care, becomes transformed by the magic that happens in that room.

## BETTY

Betty was one tough cookie. A robust woman, she towered over the other care partners. She was a very negative person and the first to find a problem with most changes. That Betty loved the residents was very apparent, but her approach focused on getting the task accomplished more than the process of doing it. She was very proud of the number of showers she could do and that her beds were generally made before the other aides' beds. She listened to the Namaste Care presentation with a dubious look on her face. She said she was a better care partner than the others but would do the job if she had to. The neighborhood had residents in all stages of dementia, so the manager assigned Betty to residents in the moderate stage of dementia.

The manager had not selected Betty to be one of the care partners assigned to work in the Namaste Care room for obvious reasons. The week after Namaste Care opened, a meeting was held to get feedback from the staff. Betty got on a roll and told management they were expecting too much from the overworked care partners. The 9:30 A.M. start time was unrealistic, and having five residents in the program was, in her words, "crazy." Other staff members jumped on board and supported Betty. They wanted management to hire more staff, which wasn't a possibility.

One day, the care partner who had been selected to lead Namaste Care called in sick. Betty was asked to fill in for her. "Absolutely not," she declared. She had not been selected at the beginning of the program, and she was perfectly happy taking care of the other residents. The manager realized that Betty might have reacted this way because she had not been selected in the first place, and her feelings were hurt.

The very wise manager asked the director of nursing (DON) to let Betty know that she thought Betty could do a very good job with programming because she knew how much Betty cared for her residents. Betty reluctantly agreed, and the next day another Namaste miracle began.

Betty arrived to begin the Namaste Care program with a small tabletop water fountain and plastic music box. At 9:30 A.M., Betty had more residents in the room than ever before. The look on her face as she was providing foot massages was that of absolute pleasure. Everyone from the administrator to the DON visited Namaste Care that day to see the "Betty miracle." It seems that Namaste Care not only enhances the lives of residents, it can do wonders for staff morale and job satisfaction.

## MARY LONGTIN

When the first Namaste Care program opened in 2003, Mary Longtin became the first Namaste Carer. Ten years later, Mary is still touching the lives of veterans and their spouses at the Vermont Veterans Home (VVH) in Bennington, VT. Christian Cosgrove, Director of Social Services at VVH, says "Mary is completely committed to making a difference in 'her' residents' lives and remains totally committed to Namaste Care. Every new resident is special, and Mary takes the time to get to know them and what would be special at this time of their lives."

Mary has touched the lives of hundreds of veterans and their spouses, recognizing that all of her special residents will spend the last days of their lives in her care. She says, "Namaste Care, even after 10 years, comforts me in knowing that I can give veterans and their families the very best personal care in a room that reminds them of home, as well as a hand to hold and shoulder to cry on. I have fond remembrances of each and every person who has touched my life. I put myself into their lives as a family member."

Once care partners get hooked on being assigned to the Namaste Care room, they tend to stay, sometime for years. Most find this slower way of providing care very satisfying. They are proud when their peers and managers come in just to see how peaceful the residents look. I have been told by harried administrators and DONs that when they are having a particularly stressful day, they come into the Namaste Care room to bask in the peacefulness of the atmosphere. Seeing the residents so calm and happy, they are reminded of why they have chosen to work in long-term care.

## NAMASTE CARE ROOM

The Namaste Care room where daily programming takes place can also be located anywhere in the facility, not in a special dementia care neighborhood, and is staffed by any care partner who expresses a desire to work with the program. Residents from the entire facility can be transported to the room by team members and become the responsibility of the Namaste Carer. In this case, a care partner might be from a neighborhood that has more residents attending the program, and one of the care partners from that neighborhood is assigned to the room. In other situations the care partner is rotated between all neighborhoods except the rehabilitation unit. I have also seen auxiliary staff take turns in the room, including restorative aides, activity assistants, and managers who sign up for an hour a week. Again, the team makes it work.

In a few instances, the slow pace in the Namaste Care room is not something care partners want to do every day, so they rotate, and each care partner has at least one day a week in the program. In some programs, care partners leading the daily program rotate, with some doing the morning activities and others the afternoon. Occasionally, the 3–11 shift does the afternoon session. Eventually one or two will shine and may decide to take on the assignment every day.

I have also heard from nurses responsible for the orientation of new employees that as part of the training for care partners, each one spends time in the Namaste Care room. Often, a new trainee expresses a desire to be a Namaste Carer after that experience. I have also been in facilities that are sites for students who would like to be certified nursing assistants or nurses. Their instructors are assigning them to the Namaste Care room as part of their training. And as the number of residents with advanced dementia grows, many facilities have more than one Namaste Care program, so the need for additional carers is challenging.

Another interesting Namaste Care model is located at Hale Nani Rehabilitation and Nursing Center in Honolulu, Hawaii, where the administrator, John J Megara, has instituted five spa-like environments that accommodate 90 residents a day who have moderate or advanced dementia. All team members participate in providing the care on a rotating basis. He recently had a staff member from the Centers for Medicare & Medicaid Services visit who was so impressed with what she saw in the Namaste Care spas she told John that if she ever had to live in a nursing home, Hale Nani would be her choice. She indicated that Namaste Care approach is exactly the type of transformational culture change the Centers for Medicare & Medicaid Services is looking to achieve.

The Hale Nani team also has a cart lovingly called Namaste à la carte that brings the program to the bedside of 50 residents who are not able or choose not to go to the spas. John has a standing order that Namaste Care happens every day. That means that if there is a shortage of staff, all team members including John and his DON, Fely Pula, and all senior management are ready and able to pitch in and ensure that the spas remain open every day. They have found that all their residents, not just those with advanced dementia, thrive from the loving touch approach to care. Mahalo (thank you), John, for teaching me another way to offer Namaste Care.

## DEDICATED NAMASTE CARER

EPOCH Senior Living has found that they need more than one Namaste Care program in their Brewster, Massachusetts, nursing facility. The original program is on the second floor, and residents from the entire facility are brought to the Namaste Care room. When the facility had more residents than space for them in the room, they started another program on the first floor of the dementia neighborhood. Although they usually hire someone with a nursing background, they selected their receptionist Averie Smith for their second program because he has a warm, nurturing personality and he loves the residents. He has done an extraordinary job, and without much of a budget but with great creativity, Averie has transformed a room that was used for family visits and staff meetings to a warm and inviting space for Namaste Care. When I visited, he had just given the women facials. Everyone looked so peaceful, their faces glistening with a beautifully scented lotion, I wanted to sit down and ask him whether I could have one. Once again, it is not about the background of the person; it's all about having the heart for this work. If the Namaste Carer position is new, a job description must be written. This company offers The Club, for residents in the middle stage of a dementing illness, and Namaste Care. They have an amazing number of deficiency-free surveys, a low staff turnover, and very low use of antipsychotic medications, which management believes justifies the additional staff.

## STAFFING THE NAMASTE CARE NEIGHBORHOOD

The population of residents with advanced dementia in nursing facilities and assisted living communities has escalated in recent years. This has resulted in some facilities developing a Namaste Care neighborhood where all team members support a palliative care approach for their residents. Often palliative care is confused with hospice care. The difference is that for the most part, hospice provides end-of-life services when a person has 6 months or less to live. Palliative care focuses on relief from pain and suffering for people with a serious illness and their families throughout the disease trajectory. Creating a special neighborhood where the goals of care are comfort and palliation provides a focus for all team members (Chapter 4).

The Namaste Care neighborhood can also be a good business decision because it provides a unique service that can be marketed to families. This can be very beneficial when a facility is trying to attract private-paying residents or when just keeping the beds full in a very competitive marketplace is challenging. The first neighborhood that I was involved with was part of the original Namaste Care program at the Vermont Veterans Home (VVH) in Bennington, Vermont. This neighborhood was created on a wing where they had several empty rooms with two or three beds in each room. At the end of the wing was a large room that could be used for the daily program. We helped to make it marketable with a new look and also offered a room (the Reagan Room) for residents who were actively dying. You will find more information about how we made the neighborhood look different in Chapter 4.

The empty beds in VVH filled quickly as families chose to move their loved ones closer to the Namaste Care room. That freed beds on the dementia care neighborhood, where they had a waiting list. Within a month the census increased significantly, making the neighborhood a good financial decision. VVH is a union facility, yet we had no problems blurring the lines of the team members' responsibilities. Families were given the option to move their loved ones to the neighborhood, so they felt in control. The result was happier families with rarely a complaint to the social workers. Family support groups emerged: a formal one that met once a month and an informal one, in which the social workers had permission to give out members' names and phone numbers to families having difficulty with the decision to move their loved ones to the neighborhood. The newly created team rose to the challenges of this ground-breaking experience, making sure music was playing in the corridors in the morning so that residents woke up to the sounds of birds chirping or soft classical sonatas. The strength of neighborhoods is the team; they will determine its success.

Recently I visited a Namaste Care neighborhood located in the Fountainview Center for Alzheimer's Disease, located in Atlanta, Georgia. Management decided that in order to provide Namaste Care to the large number of residents with advanced dementia residing in their facility, they needed to convert an entire 40-bed pavilion into a Namaste Care environment where two or three care partners would provide daily programming. The education and training director provided in-services to all departments to gain their cooperation in understanding the need for peace and quiet while programming was taking place; restricting traffic into the pavilion for a 2-hour period in the morning and afternoon was necessary. The first pavilion was so successful that another pavilion has initiated its own Namaste Care morning session for 6–12 residents. When I visited Fountainview, I could sense the pride team members had in their program. They were bubbling with excitement as they showed me a closet filled with colorful, flower-decked women's hats. I thought that someone had raided Queen Elizabeth's closet! The team members explained that something special was needed to spice up the weekends, so they schedule a tea party once a month for the women. Special care is given to applying their makeup, they wear their best dresses, and every woman who chooses to has a hat to wear for the tea. China cups are used, and families are invited to participate in the festivities. During the summer they have "beach day," when sand is brought in so that residents can wiggle their toes around in the sand, and they can bat a beach ball around and suck on flavorful popsicles. The team asked for and received permission to design T-shirts with *Namaste* and a butterfly printed on the front. This team is amazing and very proud of the palliative care they offer.

## SELECTING NAMASTE CARE
## NEIGHBORHOOD TEAM MEMBERS

The selection of team members who are able to work with residents in the advanced stage of a dementing illness is the first step in creating a Namaste Care neighborhood. Do not assume that current team members, even if they are part of an existing dementia program, will want to work in the Namaste Care neighborhood. In some dementia programs, residents who are in the advanced stage of their disease are transferred to another wing of the facility. Therefore, few residents actually die in the dementia neighborhood. Caring for residents in the moderate stages of dementia is quite different from caring for residents in the advanced or terminal stages of dementia and requires a palliative approach. The Namaste Care neighborhood is not for everyone.

It is assumed that all residents in a Namaste Care neighborhood will die within a year or two, making it imperative that team members be comfortable working in a neighborhood where death is a frequent presence. This requires a special calling. One of the important goals of Namaste Care is to provide palliative care so that the resident experiences a peaceful, pain-free, dignified death in his or her home (i.e., the nursing facility or assisted living community), surrounded by family (both relatives and staff). In addition, residents in this neighborhood are usually unable to communicate. In other neighborhoods, many elderly residents live for years. They can talk to team members, joke, express gratitude, and show love. The residents receiving Namaste Care are usually unable to express their feelings, and if a person does not have the heart for this kind of work, it can be exhausting and unrewarding if he or she does not love it.

Housekeeping staff also need to be selected for their desire to work in this neighborhood because they will be responsible for keeping the Namaste Care room clean, and that room is not a typical nursing facility room. It will be filled with items such as plants and quilts to make it look as home-like as possible, and it needs to have housekeeping staff available for cleaning between sessions. Remember that housekeepers also become close to residents and may not be comfortable working among those who are in the last stage of life.

Activity professionals who are assigned to the neighborhood may spend some time in the Namaste Care room as well as visit residents individually in their room. They will have responsibility for continually updating the seasonal and sensory items for programming in the Namaste Care room and for the Namaste Care cart used while making bedside visits in residents' rooms. They will be expected to suggest stimulating supplies and seasonal items, along with rotating music CDs and nature DVDs for the television.

Nurses and care partners selected for a Namaste Care neighborhood must be willing to provide meaningful activities and understand that the process is more important than the task itself. This is a paradigm shift for nursing team members. For example, rather than trying to give a resistant resident a shower or tub bath, the care partner gives a relaxing bed bath with soothing music playing and the scent of lavender permeating the room. If a blanket warmer is not available, use a hair dryer to warm bedding and towels.

It is sometimes difficult for nurses and care partners to change from a task-oriented approach to one more focused on process. Care partners are used to being assigned a certain number of residents to dress, groom, bathe, change, and feed. The day shift care partners are also expected to make beds, tidy the residents' rooms, and complete their assignments by the end of the shift. Added to this is the expectation that, in Namaste Care, they will be expected to talk and spend quality time with residents.

Nurses' responsibilities do not change and include calling physicians, charting, providing treatments, distributing medications, and talking with families, among a variety of other jobs that arise as the day unfolds. The Namaste Care approach requires team members to spend more time with residents and leave the other tasks until after the residents have been provided care in an unhurried way. The supervising nurses must then support the care partners as they shift their focus to this person-centered philosophy and show understanding when, for example, every bed is not made on schedule. Nurses must also be able to model care approaches and give a helping hand when needed. I love hearing that a nurse has made some beds while the care partners are busy caring for residents; this is when the team really works! Everyone on the team understands the importance of making activities of daily living meaningful.

At the Park Avenue care home located in a suburb of London, one nurse is always in the Namaste Care room providing the same gentle approach to activities of daily living as the care partners. Nurses also model how to give bed baths to residents who resist taking a shower, and the love of what they do spills over to all the team members on their floor.

Nurses, care partners, housekeeping, and activity professionals should be selected from team members who have expressed a desire to work with residents who are in the last stage of their illness. As part of the introductory in-service that explains how a Namaste Care neighborhood will function, team members are asked to talk with their supervisor if they are interested in working there. They are then interviewed by the person supervising Namaste Care.

Care partners who express a desire to work with Namaste Care residents are interviewed by the charge nurse to make sure they have the necessary clinical skills. The neighborhood manager, if that person is not a nurse, may be included in the interview. During the interview, staff members are informed of the expectations of Namaste Care and assured that if after working on the neighborhood they decide this is not what they enjoy, they will be transferred to another neighborhood without any negative repercussions. Interviews also provide an opportunity to ask staff members how they feel about their work. Many care partners have worked in long-term care for many years and may have lost the enthusiasm they once had for the job.

## JOHN

> John had been a care partner in the same facility for more than 15 years. During the interview, he pleaded with the charge nurse to let him work in the Namaste Care neighborhood. He said, "I've forgotten why I started doing this work in the first place. I think Namaste Care will help me regain that feeling I used to have. At the end of the day, I can go home and feel good about what I have accomplished that day. Now, I go home exhausted and think of everything I didn't get to."

## SUPERVISION

Namaste Care is usually under the overall supervision of the assistant director of nursing because it is primarily a nursing program, and the DON is overwhelmed with other responsibilities. If it is located in a Dementia Special Care or Namaste Care neighborhood, the manager usually provides supervision of the daily program. In the Atlanta situation, the nurse assigned to education and training supervises the pavilion. I have also seen successful programs where the activity professional provides supervision, with a nurse monitoring the clinical aspects of the daily activities. The Namaste Care checklist is a helpful tool for ongoing supervision and can be found in Appendix D. It is always a good idea to ask the nurse in charge of infection control to make a visit at least once a month to make sure all those procedures are in place.

Namaste Care supervisors are also responsible for helping Namaste Carers and care partners feel appreciated. They have a difficult job, often a thankless one. Working day after day with residents who cannot carry on a conversation, say "thank you," or remember their caregivers' names is not easy. Resident deaths are a fact of life, yet there is often little or no time to grieve. Families are another variable that may not always be easy to deal with. Some family members direct the frustration and anger evoked by the disease toward the nurses and care partners. Just as the residents need special care, so too do the staff members.

Verbal praise is an absolute must for members of the Namaste Care team. They should be greeted with the same respect and care with which they greet residents every day. Gestures such as hugging, if appropriate, asking about their families, and letting them know that the team is glad to have them back after a few days off help them feel valued. Offering simple pleasantries makes such a difference. Fresh doughnuts or other goodies are a nice way to say "thank you." When the supervisor does something personal, such as cooking something special for the team, the bond between team members is strengthened. Namaste Care is not only about a special way of caring for residents, it is about caring for all team members.

A kind word from management, especially the administrator or DON, does wonders for team members' self-esteem. Timely evaluations, especially those that include a raise, show respect for staff members. Long-term care workers do not make a great deal of money, so even a small raise can make a difference to them.

Families often tell the charge nurse how happy they are with a care partner but do not tell the care partner. Family members should be asked to take the time to personally thank Namaste Carers who do a particularly good job or have done something special for them or their loved one. Any written thank-you letter should be posted on the neighborhood. If a staff person has been mentioned by name, the letter should be copied for the individual and the human resources director.

## ASSIGNING SPECIFIC RESPONSIBILITIES

Namaste Care is usually led by a care partner, with support from the activity department. The Namaste Carer assigned for the day opens the Namaste Care room after breakfast and stays in the room until lunch. Other team members should come in periodically to relieve the Namaste Carer for breaks and lunch. If the Namaste Carer has been hired just for the daily program, he or she may also help feed breakfast and lunch to the residents in the neighborhood.

After the residents have had lunch and been toileted, the Namaste Care room reopens. When I first started the program, the afternoon program usually had fewer residents because some residents take a nap during this time. Now they may be completely full because more residents need Namaste Care than can fit into the room for the morning session. In that instance some residents attend the morning session and others the afternoon session. I have also spent more time talking to nursing about the residents' quality of life when they attend Namaste Care instead of going to their rooms for a nap. They can sleep in the Namaste Care room where they will not be alone and can hear the music and voices and smell the lavender. They spend enough time in their beds because most are put to bed right after dinner. The exception would be when a resident is at risk for skin problems. These residents need to be transferred from their chair to the bed and positioned properly to lower the potential of skin breakdown. After an hour or two, they can be taken back to the Namaste Care room.

If there is not a special Namaste Carer who is dedicated to the room, when the afternoon shift arrives, one care partner is assigned to the room until the residents are taken to the dining area for dinner. The Namaste Care room could also be opened in the evening, with one care partner in the room while the others are getting residents ready for bed.

If the Namaste Carer is a separate position, typical hours are 9:00 A.M. to 5:00 P.M. This leaves a half hour in the morning for gathering supplies and getting the room ready for the day, another half hour of quiet time before lunch to dispose of soiled laundry and refresh linens and other supplies, and a final half hour at the end of the day to work on charting and get the room ready for the next day.

## HANDLING STAFFING SHORTAGES

Staffing shortages are a reality in the long-term care business, requiring supervisors to be resourceful. This is when all team members join together to make Namaste Care happen 7 days a week. Although everyone may not be able to do some activities that they have to be qualified to do, such as offering beverages (regulations differ from state to state and country to country), it is more important to have the room open and just have a team member sit beside a resident and hold his or her hand. Creative ways to staff Namaste Care in emergencies include the following:

- Put out an alert that staffing is needed and ask team members to sign up for at least a 30-minute shift. All team members have had a basic orientation and been given suggestions on providing some of the meaningful activities, or they are encouraged to simply play music and talk to the residents. Managers will have to approve staff leaving their usual assigned duties. It's incredible to see team members whom you would have never expected to enjoy Namaste Care shine. In one unforgettable experience, a dietary aide signed up for a 30-minute shift. She asked her manager what she could do, and the answer was "do what is in your heart," so this young woman began to sing, astonishing everyone. No one knew she had such a beautiful voice. Another surprise was a receptionist who startled everyone when he spent his 30 minutes fixing the women's hair. Not many people knew he had been a hairdresser. I happened to be there when this happened, and as he left the room I thanked him for filling in. His response was, "I know I got more out of this than the residents. I really felt useful. Thank you."

- Schedule the nursing staff to come in for short periods to offer beverages and check on the residents' comfort and safety.

- Ask activity professionals to replace individual visits with spending part of their day in the Namaste Care room.

- Call volunteers who have been oriented to provide Namaste Care activities. Even when in an emergency situation, such as a shortage of team members, they are never to be left in the room without a team member present.

Another idea that adds extra hands in the Namaste Care room is to assign staff members who are on limited or light duty, who cannot carry out the tasks of their regular position yet have been released by their physician to return to work.

## PATTY

Patty was a dedicated care partner who did not think Namaste Care was for her. She loved her work with the residents, and the residents loved her. She had surgery on her knee and was out of work for a month. Her physician gave her the go-ahead to work again but ordered her to be off of her feet for the majority of the day—not realistic for a care partner who is on the go all day. She was placed on light duty and assigned to the Namaste Care room, where with a low chair that wheeled around, provided by the rehab department, she fell in love with the program, and when she returned to her regular duties as a care partner, she checked out at the end of her shift and spent time in the Namaste Care room as a volunteer.

## TIM

Tim was a care partner whom everyone dreaded having assigned to their neighborhood. He had been employed in a unionized building for several years and knew how far he could push the envelope without getting written up. He certainly knew that the supervisors didn't like him and, as a result, he became even more difficult to work with. One day he was on light duty, and it was apparent that he planned to do as little as he could get away with. The nursing supervisor had other plans and assigned him to the Namaste Care room. Everyone held their breath waiting for him to explode with anger, his usual reaction when he didn't like something. To their surprise, Tim was inspired! He shaved the men, massaged feet, and joked with the women; the room shined! No one could believe it; one by one, managers trooped down to the Namaste Care room to see this transformation and congratulate Tim on doing a great job. Positive reinforcement made him very pleased with himself. He said it was the best day he had experienced in many years—Namaste Care magic at work again.

## RETAINING STAFF

The turnover of care partners in long-term care is very high. I have worked in some homes where the turnover of care partners is more than 100%. For human resources, it is a never-ending cycle of recruitment and orientation; staff members work a few months and leave, and the process repeats itself. Attracting and retaining good staff is difficult. The Pioneer Network has found that nursing facilities that have embraced culture change have a significantly lower turnover rate than the national average. These facilities have eliminated overtime, decreased use of temporary agency staff, and lowered compensation costs. Administrators report that staff members feel better about their jobs and want to be a part of something fresh and new.

Namaste Care fits in with the culture-change movement, because it is about person-directed care and the rights of residents to continue to be involved in life for as long as they live and to be honored and cared for in a respectful manner. The quality of life residents experience extends to the team members who care for them; they also feel as if their quality of life improves because they like or love their jobs. They are part of a caring group of people who make a positive difference in their residents' lives. Because all Namaste Care team members are involved in decision making as the program evolves, they feel empowered to suggest changes. When staff members feel as if they are valued, turnover is significantly lower.

Unfortunately, we live in a media-defined world, and the gorier the story, the more press it receives. Those of us in long-term care know better; we see thousands of moments every day when staff go way above and beyond the call of duty to make their residents' world a little brighter. From a team member who fixes ethnic food to tempt someone who is not eating very well, to one who comes in on her day off to sit by the bedside of a favorite resident who is dying, these millions of moments help to define long-term care.

When I was a child, I had no athletic talent whatsoever. The kids in my neighborhood loved to play ball, and we would organize games after school and on weekends. I missed the ball quite often; more than the three misses that were allowed. Then I would plead for a "do over" that would give me one more chance to hit that darn ball. Namaste Care ensures quality at the end of life because, as we know, there is no "do over" for our residents.

# CHAPTER 4

# The Namaste Care Setting

Where thou art, that is home.

EMILY DICKINSON

The Namaste Care™ daily program can be offered in a variety of settings as a dedicated room or room that is also used for other purposes, such as dining or activities. The setting needs to look and feel comfortable to support the Namaste Care program. If the facility is part of a large chain, the corporation's professional designers can be used to help create the ambiance of the room. A facility might also have a budget for hiring an interior designer. It is important to make sure this design professional knows the regulations for health care settings, understands the physiological changes and special needs of residents with dementia (Brawley, 2006), and is familiar with the Namaste Care daily programming. This year, I had the good fortune to work with professional designers for Arden Courts who had health care experience and took the time to learn about Namaste Care. Their team of designers visited one of the first programs we implemented so they could see for themselves what changes needed to be made in the living room to support and enhance the program. The result was a Namaste Care room that was practical, containing the supplies and equipment we needed, yet beautiful, with an electric fireplace that added a special homey touch to each room. A shade with beautiful pictures painted on one side could be pulled down to cover a half wall, and a drape installed at the large open entrance to the room could be tied back when the program was not in session. These professional touches eliminated distractions while the program was taking place. (More information on working with these professional designers can be found in Chapter 4.)

Most of the time, however, there is no money for these services. An excellent resource to use is the maintenance director, who can give advice on regulations regarding fire ratings for fabrics and rules for a safe egress from the room. Most often the Namaste Care team members are creative and spaces become transformed into comfortable and comforting, home-like settings.

Programming can be offered anywhere that there is a space to gather residents in the presence of others so that they are no longer isolated. Whatever the allocation of space, small or large, giving it a different appearance from the rest of the facility helps residents, their families, and staff members know that they are in a special place. Making the space look different also helps with marketing it as a new program. A coat of paint can work wonders!

Most spaces in a long-term care facility have challenges, whether it is turning an empty resident's room into a homey-looking Namaste Care room or making a large area look warm and cozy. Actually, working on very little money is a specialty of mine, and I am often dubbed the Queen of Wal-Mart décor! When the team works with a limited budget and can still make remarkable transformations in challenging spaces just by being resourceful and imaginative, the team spirit grows as the room begins to change. At times I believe the excitement generated by these preparations makes the program a success before it opens.

It is important to always keep in mind that Namaste Care is not about the room itself but about what transpires in the room. As I mentioned in the previous chapter about who actually provides the daily programming, this is not about money; it's about having the heart to make it happen. A great example of this was with the first Namaste Care program in Australia, where there was no un-used space for a dedicated room.

## SYDNEY, AUSTRALIA

I was speaking about Namaste Care at a conference for the School of Nursing at the University of Western Sydney, Australia. Several months before the conference, I was on a call with the organizers discussing details of my time there. One of the people on the planning commit-tee mentioned how nice it would be to actually have a program for people to see. And without thinking, I blurted out that if they could find a care home that after reading my book wanted to do it, I could have one up in 4 days. Of course, I never thought that would happen, but I underestimated school research director Esther Chang, a deceptively tiny woman who is a dynamo and gets things done. The next thing I knew, a care home decided they would love to have the first Namaste Care program in Australia. And before I knew it, I was in Sydney mak-ing Namaste Care happen in 4 days. The only space I could find that was big enough was a section of one dining room that jutted out in a strange angle from the main dining area and was used just for feeding a few residents. I was assured that the feeding could take place in a small room near the nurses' station, and we could use that space. It was located by the entrance to the dining room, so the distraction of having everyone pass by was a problem.

The night before we opened, the very clever and talented adminis-trator bought some material and sewed a curtain to separate it from the main dining room. Early on the morning of the grand opening, the maintenance worker hung a cable from one side of the opening to the other. He then attached the curtain with hooks that allowed it to be pulled over to the side when we brought residents into the room and when closed would shield the room from distractions. I found a couple of tall plants that I placed at the opening to make it look presentable. In 1 hour we transformed the room by covering old geri-chairs found in the basement with pretty floral sheets, hanging pictures on the wall, placing live plants on the window sills, and putting little vases of fresh flowers on small tables scattered around the room. The program opened that morning to looks of disbelief from staff and families, and we had ourselves a Namaste Care room.

## CREATING A HOME-LIKE DEDICATED NAMASTE CARE ROOM

The Namaste Care room is a space designated for daily programming. Ideally this is a room that is dedicated to Namaste Care programming and can be secured when not in use. In this case, it can be decorated with an array of antique objects, real plants, and other items that add warmth and character to the room yet would not be a problem for a wandering resident who might decide to eat a plant or to "shop" by taking items from the room. Several easy steps can guarantee a restful, cheerful environment for not a lot of money.

The first step is deciding on the color of the room. Unless the room has recently been painted, repainting it in a different color will give it a fresh, new look. I have found that soft pastel colors work the best in yellow, peach, green, or blue and if possible with a matching wallpaper border, preferably one with a floral print. This begins to create the soft, soothing environment that is Namaste Care.

If getting the room painted would be difficult for the maintenance staff, recruit volunteers to paint and hang a border. Decorating the Namaste Care room is a perfect project for a service organization or generous benefactor. Painting and hanging the border is a one-weekend project with immediate results. Volunteers like to be able to make a visible difference. My first job was in a very old building that I thought desperately needed to be redecorated. In one year just asking various service clubs, military clubs such as the Veterans of Foreign Wars, and churches, we repainted the entire facility. The work was done on weekends when volunteers had more time and less was going on in the facility. Small plaques thanking the various organizations were located outside each of the rooms.

Redecorating the Namaste Care room also provides an opportunity for fundraising. Some benefactors prefer to donate money rather than time and labor. Consider dedicating the Namaste Care room to the memory of a loved one of some of your biggest benefactors.

Once the room is painted, the next step is to furnish it and add home-like touches. Here are some easy and affordable options:

- Look in facility storage closets and basements for pictures and furniture left behind by former residents.

- Visit Goodwill or used furniture stores for tables, cabinets, lamps, and other interesting pieces of furniture that will help to make the room look like a living room. Be on the lookout for buffets, as they are good storage pieces. Gently used furniture can be made more presentable with furniture polish that covers scratches. Stripping and staining old furniture is time consuming, but the finished piece can be a wonderful reminder of furniture that residents have owned in the past. You may have success asking family volunteers to help refinish used furniture. Use doilies on tables to hide scratches and provide an old-fashioned look.

- Check out garage or yard sales, called rumble sales in the United Kingdom, for furniture and old items such as sewing baskets, pieces of quilts that can be framed, and pieces of embroidery and lace.

- Purchase pictures and artwork at discount stores such as Wal-Mart or Target in the clearance section.

- Use wall stickers and art that have quotes, are easy to install, and can be moved.

- Ask for donations of plants or plant cuttings, and recruit a plant volunteer to keep them healthy. The local garden club may assist with filling the room with live plants and flowers.

- Hang wind chimes and brightly colored sun catchers in the windows.

- Install a bird feeder outside the window.

- Ask families for pictures of the residents and arrange them around the room.

- Place a portable waterfall near a wall; they are inexpensive and make a lovely sound.

Before any electrical appliances are used, such as table lamps, blenders, and CD players, make sure that the maintenance department checks them for safety problems. They can attach a sticker with the date of inspection so that surveyors and the fire marshal know that they have been approved.

Storing supplies in the room or space used for Namaste Care eliminates the time needed to set the room up every day. If a resident's room is being used for the program, install shelves in the closet for supplies and add a lock if needed. Use a rod in the closet to hang large bags for storing the individual quilts and blankets that are used each day to wrap around residents to provide warmth and comfort. Wardrobes can be used for storage and can be secured. Also, because so many people have flat-screen television sets now, television cabinets that were used to hold the old-style television sets are now being discarded, and they make perfect storage units. When the room can be secured, colorful plastic or fabric storage containers are attractive enough so that they do not need to be hidden and become part of the room's décor.

If the room can be secured, a kitchen nook is a wonderful feature to add to the Namaste Care room. A sink, small refrigerator, and microwave are practical and help to create the home-like feeling of the room. Hanging old kitchen utensils on the wall and placing old-fashioned magnets on the refrigerator, using antique dish towels, hanging colorful aprons on hooks, and having a cookie jar and bread box on the counter help to establish a country kitchen. I just Googled "old fashioned kitchen items," and some fun and inexpensive web sites popped up. In one nursing facility the maintenance worker found a kitchen cabinet that looked like wood in the clearance section of a building supply store. He installed it in a corner of the room, and we placed a microwave and cookie jar on it; a small refrigerator stood beside the counter. For very little expense, this area became a kitchenette where the food and beverages we needed for the daily programs were stored.

One of the first programs I implemented for EPOCH Senior Living was in an empty two-person resident room.

## TRANSFORMING A RESIDENT ROOM

A resident room was painted the same color and had the same window treatments as all the other rooms in the neighborhood. We wanted to create a different look without making any changes that would cause problems if the room needed to be restored to a resident room. All the furniture was removed, and the room was painted a soft yellow. A flowered border was hung, and the room sprang to life.

The staff went on a hunting expedition in storage closets and in the basement. They found some small tables and paintings that had been donated to the facility by the families of deceased residents. An inexpensive plant rack painted a soft green was placed in one corner; it did not take up much space and added some color to the room. Families and residents donated their extra plants to the room, and we purchased African violets for the window sill. These flowers are easy to care for and bloom most of the time. A bird feeder was attached to the outside window, providing enjoyment for several residents.

We discovered an old stereo system, the kind that looked like a piece of furniture popular in the seventies. It no longer worked and was not practical to fix, but we cleaned and polished it, and it became a useful piece of furniture. We covered it with a lace scarf, then arranged pictures, a basket of lollipops, and a plant on it. No one could recognize what it had been in its former life.

The room had two disconnected call bells mounted on the wall, which made the room look institutional. An inexpensive patchwork quilt was purchased, sprayed with fire-retardant spray, and hung over the fixtures with double-faced tape. The result was an inexpensive yet attractive way to hide the call bell system. Art for the walls and other interesting knickknacks came from the marketing department, which donated some items from the stash of decorating pieces used for model and respite rooms.

A private bathroom with a tub, toilet, and sink was already located in the room. Because no one was going to take a bath during Namaste Care, a pretty shower curtain was hung to hide a storage area for supplies created by placing shelving in the bathtub. Residents would not be toileted in the room, so additional shelves were placed over the toilet. Pretty towels and a few pictures of old-fashioned bathrooms converted this resident bathroom into a practical yet pretty room.

Lounge chairs were not in the budget, but some unused geri-chairs were found in the basement. Their trays were removed, quilts were hung over the chairs, and cute pillows were placed on the seats to help hide the very institutional look of the chairs. In a few weeks and with little cost, this room was transformed.

It is amazing what can be done with great spirit and little money. It was fun to see the looks on the faces of staff and family members when they saw the transformation. If they only knew how we did it! Very quickly the room filled, and more residents than could be accommodated were identified as needing Namaste Care. A larger space was found so that the program could grow, and the original space was restored to a resident room. Using a resident room on a temporary basis meant that the beds did not have to be decertified, and the room with its new paint and border was desirable and quickly filled.

The simple placement of furniture and accessories can make a difference in how the room looks. For instance, adding a needlepoint pillow and afghan to a rocking chair placed beside a floor lamp creates a small, comfortable niche that family members gravitate toward. The room should have a few chairs for families and a resident who just wanders in to sit for a while. It's also good to have lounge chairs or place residents in the room in small settings not in a circle. Perhaps a few chairs can be placed in front of the television. Two chairs can be angled to face a window so that residents can see outside. In Michigan a flock of swans live in a pond outside the Namaste Care room. When I visited, mamma swan was proudly sitting on her nest, much to the delight of the residents peering through the window. Bird feeders can be located outside the window, and hummingbird feeders can be stuck to the windows.

A Namaste Care room that has a circle of chairs looks very institutional, and I think it looks sad. Stand at the door and try to see the room as if it is a new experience for you. Does it look as comfortable and home-like as possible? If not, change it around so that it does. If you are not working with a designer, marketing staff often have an eye for arranging furniture.

When Namaste Care team members have a vision for how the room should look, they often will find gems while shopping. In one facility, a rehabilitation aide discovered a buffet while she was browsing in a local Goodwill store. After it was polished and most of the scratches covered, it looked quite presentable. The drawers were kept open to show old lace tablecloths, colorful shawls, and other sensory items used for programming. It was a beautiful addition to the Namaste Care room. Old, used furniture pieces are perfect additions that help create a lived-in look and in some cases are more inviting than expensive new purchases.

When we were assembling the Namaste Care room at the Vermont Veterans Home (VVH) in Bennington, Vermont, their administrator allowed any team member to buy an item for the room as long as it was under $25 and they had a receipt. This encouraged the team to feel a part of creating the room. Many of the team donated pictures, quilts, and antiques just because they wanted to.

## A DUAL-PURPOSE ROOM

In some facilities, the Namaste Care room is used for other purposes, most often as the dining room. In this case, it is not feasible to equip the room with many of the home-like features of a room totally dedicated to Namaste Care, such as live plants, afghans on chairs, and antique items. It would be too difficult to keep these items in the room, especially in a dementia care neighborhood where residents may wander in and claim them as their own.

However, dual-purpose rooms can still look warm and friendly. Lounge chairs provide comfortable seating for ambulatory residents or those who are easily transferred from a wheelchair and can sit safely in them. A secured storage area is necessary if supplies are kept in the room; if this is not possible, a rolling cart with all the supplies needed for the day can be taken out of the room when Namaste Care programming ends. Silk plants and flowers are used rather than live plants for residents' safety.

Although dual-purpose rooms are not the best option, you can always make do with what you have, and the room can be staged for the program.

### EPOCH SENIOR HEALTHCARE OF NORTON, MASSACHUSETTS

This facility is the oldest purpose-built nursing home in Massachusetts and did not have space for a dedicated Namaste Care room. The wing we selected for the Namaste Care program had just one day room that was also where residents ate meals. The maintenance staff repainted the room a soft blue and hung a border of pastel flowers at the top of all walls. Blinds that were constantly getting bent and broken by residents were replaced with soft white lace curtains. We placed shelves on the walls, high enough so that residents could not reach them, and filled them with old-fashioned knickknacks. They already had a television set and DVD player that we could use for nature videos.

A discarded television cabinet became a storage unit for supplies, and the administrator approved the purchase of six comfortable lounge chairs that we used for our program. They were pushed close to the walls, making room for the dining tables. When Namaste Care was not in session, residents and families enjoyed sitting in them when they were visiting.

Staging the room became an art for Namaste Carer Margaret Silva. After breakfast and lunch, the room was emptied of residents and housekeeping cleaned the floors. Margaret pushed some of the dining tables to the corners of the room, and others became part of the program and were staged with tablecloths and items such as a tea set and framed pictures of the residents. On one day when I was visiting Margaret had fresh lilacs in vases on them; another day she sprinkled silk rose petals on the tables. Before the program officially began, Margaret gathered supplies, switched on a diffuser with lavender-scented oil, played calming music, and dimmed the lights, and the room took on a new personality. Then Margaret opened the door to welcome residents, and they felt as if they were in a different place. She hung a sign that welcomes people to come into the room because the door is closed during the program.

In other situations, family rooms are used during the day for Namaste Care, and in the evening they become a place for family visits. The rooms have a closet where supplies can be stored and have comfortable lounge chairs so the dual use is easy to accomplish.

## NAMASTE CARE NEIGHBORHOOD

From a business perspective, offering a Namaste Care neighborhood has the potential to increase census and attract private-paying residents. Before this decision is made, a need assessment is conducted. An evaluation of the current dementia program is a good first step. Assess the physical and cognitive status of the residents currently in the dementia program and residents on other neighborhoods to determine the need for a dedicated advanced care neighborhood. Then, determine the market for attracting residents with moderate dementia who would be needed to fill the beds of residents with advanced dementia who would be transferred from the special dementia care neighborhood. This would be just an estimate because no one would be made to move.

Increased revenue from a special program is another financial consideration. Special Care Dementia neighborhoods usually charge a higher daily rate for private-paying residents than other neighborhoods. Whether for profit or not for profit, the reality of the long-term care business is that it must make money or at least break even. Most states are faced with cuts in both Medicaid and Medicare funds, and that is not likely to change in the next few years. And assisted living communities are keeping residents longer, so the number of private-paying residents looking for nursing facility placement has decreased.

With the number of people with Alzheimer's disease growing at an astounding rate and with no cure on the horizon, making dementia care a specialty may be a good financial decision. This may also help to attract private-paying residents. Furthermore, offering two programs, one for residents with moderate dementia and one for advanced, can help position your facility as providing excellent and unique services. So making Namaste Care a profit center may be a good business decision.

From a quality-of-care perspective, a Namaste Care neighborhood can have its own dedicated staff, selected for their desire to specialize in working with residents in the advanced stage of dementia. Staff members who choose to work in special neighborhoods are usually extremely dedicated to their work and proud that they are part of a unique program. This was certainly true for the first Namaste Care program, which started as a dedicated neighborhood in a skilled nursing facility in Bennington, Vermont.

## VERMONT VETERANS HOME

The VVH shows how a dedicated Namaste Care neighborhood can be successful in many ways. From a business standpoint, it increased census by freeing beds in the dementia care neighborhood, where they had a waiting list. With the permission of their families, residents with advanced dementia were moved to an adjoining Namaste Care neighborhood where there were empty beds. The facility also experienced an increase in referrals from discharge planners and hospice staff who were working with families who had loved ones with advanced dementia.

Surveyors loved Namaste Care. They even asked permission to recommend that other nursing facilities in the state visit VVH to learn how to improve care for residents with advanced dementia. The neighborhood also generated positive publicity for the facility through conference presentations and articles published in professional journals.

The Namaste Care neighborhood was part of a 17-bed wing divided by a central nurses' station. Fire doors were at the entrance to the neighborhood, and the neighborhood had the typical double-loaded corridor found in many nursing facilities. The Namaste Care room was located at the end of the corridor. The neighborhood had one private room; the remaining rooms were for double occupancy. The social worker's office was located on the neighborhood, as was a utility room and shower area with toilets. There was no budget for decorating the neighborhood, so costs had to be kept low.

The institutional look of the corridor was changed by painting it a soft taupe and hanging a border. Walls were transformed with artwork from the local community. The facility initiated a Gifts of Love program intended to encourage local artists to donate original works of art for the neighborhood. A letter describing the program and asking for donations was sent to previous benefactors, artists, and anyone else who might contribute to funding Namaste Care. The letter was also published in the local newspaper as a public relations initiative. Several artists donated work; other benefactors donated money, which enabled management to purchase an adjustable double bed, bed linens, and carpeting for the private room that eventually became the Reagan Room. Mary Longtin, the original Namaste Carer, is an artist, and she helped to group pictures and other decorative items on the walls, including the Chinese symbols for peace and tranquility, a small quilt, and pictures of the local landscape. The corridor was transformed from an institutional-looking space to one that was warm and peaceful—no easy feat with a very limited budget. When it was finished, Namaste Care team members found ways to disguise laundry carts and other unsightly items. They took great pride in how the neighborhood looked.

Regulations required the name of each resident to be posted outside his or her room, so VVH staff purchased bulletin boards in a soft taupe fabric that had ribbons to hold memorabilia as well as the resident's name and room number. These were sprayed with flame retardant to satisfy fire regulations. Families were asked to provide copies (not originals) of pictures, as well as greeting cards or items that reflected the residents' past interests. One family tucked the resident's favorite recipe cards on her bulletin board. In this facility, all the men and some of the women were veterans, so each bulletin board had an insignia showing the branch of service under which they had served. Small flags were tucked in the ribbons. Using bulletin boards that were beautiful yet practical made the long corridor look less institutional.

In this neighborhood, fire doors were closed (but not secured) to lower the noise level. Soft music played in the corridor throughout the day. One team member was designated the lead care partner and assumed responsibility for turning on the music and ensuring that one care partner was always on the neighborhood. Doors were kept open while residents were transported to the dining area and at night when fewer staff were assigned to the neighborhood.

A shower room was located on the neighborhood. It, too, received a makeover. Painting it blue, hanging pretty shower curtains and crisp white curtains, placing silk flowers on the window sills, and hanging old-fashioned bathroom pictures helped to make the room pretty. With all the changes on this neighborhood, anyone entering the doors knew immediately that it was a special place.

Namaste Care is about providing special programming and offering unique services to residents with advanced dementia and their families. All can take place in a variety of spaces. The areas dedicated to Namaste Care should be as quiet as possible, with no overhead paging or other institutional sounds. Call bells may be changed to produce a chime sound or play a tune to support the home-like environment of the neighborhood or the room (Calkins, 2005). It is amazing how making the spaces comfortable and home-like and reducing the noise level can help to create a calming atmosphere. Namaste Care happens through Namaste Care team members' dedication and willingness to go the extra mile to make the dream of providing top-quality, compassionate care to their dying residents a reality.

## ADDITIONAL DEDICATED NAMASTE CARE SPACES

As the Bennington Namaste Care neighborhood began to expand, team members began to look at all the spaces on the neighborhood to see how they could be used for Namaste Care.

### Family Room

Having a room for families to use is a valuable feature of a Namaste Care neighborhood. In this case, the social worker's office was on the Namaste Care neighborhood, and she readily agreed to move so that a family room could be created. A donation paid for a sleep sofa for family members who wanted to stay overnight. Another family donated antique furniture that made the room look like an old-fashioned living room. A small table and chairs were added so that the room could be used for care plan meetings for the residents on the neighborhood. Family conferences could be held in the room as well as private visits with social workers and the clergy. Some families also just use such a room to take a break from sitting with their family member.

### The Reagan Room

We realized that when residents were actively dying, and they were in a double room, the families had little opportunity for privacy. The administrator and board of directors approved the use of the only private room on the Namaste Care neighborhood for that purpose. It was named the Reagan Room, in memory of former president Ronald Reagan, and its impact was fast and remarkable. Families were so grateful to have this private space to use during such a difficult time that they began to give donations to the Reagan Room. Many also asked their friends and family members to give donations in lieu of flowers in memory of their loved one. So the room was an instant success in many ways.

Families whose loved one was actively dying were given the choice of letting the resident stay in his or her room or move to the Reagan Room. Families on the Namaste Care neighborhood were given priority, but the room was also offered to families whose loved one lived anywhere in the facility. Most families chose to have their loved one moved because of the privacy it afforded the family. We worried that it would be viewed as the death room. However, this was not the case, perhaps because we decorated it to look beautiful and because of the positive reactions from staff and families.

The room was painted a soft peach, carpeting was laid, and blinds were hung on the large window. Donations made possible the purchase of a dresser and a motorized double bed. This allowed Namaste Carers to give care easily because the bed could be repositioned. What we did not anticipate was how the double bed allowed spouses to lie next to their loved ones as they were dying. Beautiful bedding was purchased for the bed. Two quilted bedspreads (so that one could be laundered while the other was being used), matching pillow shams, and peach-colored sheets and pillowcases helped to create a very home-like bedroom.

If you work in a nursing facility, you know that lost laundry is an unfortunate reality. Team members cringed when we showed them the beautiful linens we purchased for the room. Everyone was anticipating that they would be laundered to death or disappear. That was never a problem because we went directly to the laundry department and asked for help. We explained about the Reagan Room and invited them to visit. We showed the laundry staff the bedding we had purchased and asked them how we could keep track of the items and keep them looking beautiful. They hand stitched a personalized name tag and gave us a special laundry bag for the items in this room. They were proud of their contribution to the room. We also met with the housekeeping staff. After we explained the room's purpose and our need to keep it ready at a moment's notice, they took special pride in polishing the furniture and keeping the room clean and in good order.

As soon as a resident was moved to the room, we transferred his or her mementos, pictures, and various other personal items. A box of items such as silk flowers and pictures for the bureau were gathered to keep the room looking personal even when it was unoccupied.

A reclining lounge chair ensured that families could be comfortable if they were sitting in the room or wanted to sleep. The

Reagan Room had its own bathroom, which was painted and decorated with a pretty wallpaper border, matching shower curtains, towels, face cloths, bathmat, and wastebasket. Pictures were hung, and this formerly boring beige room was transformed to an attractive bathroom for families. Medical supplies were hidden from sight behind the shower curtain, so it was a practical space also.

The Reagan Room continues to provide a beautiful place for families of residents who are dying. The double bed was one of the best decisions we made, as it has made such a difference for families spending their last hours with a loved one. Joan, the wife of one resident, tells the story of her last night together with her husband.

*JOAN*

Joan received a telephone call one evening from the charge nurse. Her husband, Jeffery, was not doing well, and she might like to come to the facility. She dressed quickly and drove to the facility as fast as she could. Joan had been living with her husband's Alzheimer's disease for many years, and although she recognized that he was declining, she just didn't believe he was dying. He had a cold, but surely he would recover as he had so many times in the past. When she arrived at the facility and saw Jeffery, she realized that his condition was more serious than she originally thought. The charge nurse took her to the family room and told her that she may want to call the rest of the family, as Jeffery's condition was quite serious. Joan was offered the use of the Reagan Room. She broke down in tears and struggled with the decision to move Jeffery. With gentle prodding from the charge nurse, she agreed to try it. He could always be moved back to his room if he got better. Joan says it was the best decision she could have made. For the remainder of the night, she lay next to Jeffery and held him in her arms. She talked to him about their life together and recalled memories from the day they met. As the sun was rising, she finished her story and Jeffery slipped away. Joan feels that somehow Jeffery heard her, and the closeness offered by the double bed made the passing an intimate experience.

Staff members have commented on how a special aura permeates the Reagan Room. Since the Reagan Room opened, it has created a haven for hundreds of families saying goodbye to their loved ones.

## MATTHEW'S STORY

Matthew was one of the first residents to be moved to the Namaste Care neighborhood. Although it was a difficult decision for his wife, Celia, to leave staff that she had grown close to, she was grateful that his room would be close to the Namaste Care room. He was in the Namaste Care neighborhood when his physical condition worsened.

Nursing identified Matthew as entering the actively dying stage 4 days before his death. He was difficult to rouse, was very lethargic, and developed a fever. The charge nurse called the physician, who agreed that comfort care should be continued and the fever treated with acetaminophen. The charge nurse and neighborhood director approached Celia to see whether she would feel comfortable moving Matthew to the Reagan Room. She had been watching the changes in the room and loved what had been created, so she agreed to have her husband moved. Matthew's personal pictures and other mementos were also moved to the room. Music selected by Celia filled the room, and she decided that Matthew would enjoy having the drapes opened because he always enjoyed seeing the beauty of nature. Namaste Care team members checked on Matthew several times each hour to assess his condition, take care of his personal needs, and make sure Celia had food and beverages available and that she was comfortable being alone with Matthew.

He was kept comfortable with morphine and appeared to be very peaceful. Matthew's children arrived shortly after he was moved to the Reagan Room, so Celia always had at least one family member with her. The family was offered food and beverages and overnight accommodations in the facility's guest room. When Matthew seemed to rally on the third day, his children returned to their homes in Massachusetts. As soon as they left, his condition worsened; it appeared that Matthew did not want to die with his children present. The Namaste Care team members then stepped in to provide support and comfort for Celia. She was never alone for the last hours of Matthew's life. In the privacy of the Reagan Room, Celia was able to face the death of her beloved husband with a few chosen staff members who were with her until Matthew took his last breath.

# CHAPTER 5

# The Namaste Care Day

Activities are meaningful when they reflect
a person's interests and lifestyle, are enjoyable
to the person, help the person to feel useful,
and provide a sense of belonging.

KATHY LAURENHUE

Namaste Care™ is a 7-day-a-week program that is offered to residents who no longer can or choose not to participate in planned activities. The Namaste Care approach has the potential to encompass many aspects of residents' lives, not just the daily program of activities. It can be an around-the-clock way of providing care that uses comforting approaches and fills each resident's day with opportunities to engage in meaningful activities. Team members interact with residents throughout their waking hours and honor them as unique individuals. Each resident's day is filled with planned and unplanned activities that include the hundreds of interactions with team members that provide the opportunity for everyone to touch and talk with him or her. These are moments for team members to experience meaningful connections as they see residents' responses to their efforts. Team members understand that residents with advanced dementia will communicate with their eyes, body language, and sounds because their ability to speak is severely impaired.

The Namaste Care approach is based on the "power of loving touch" and reframes the process of providing activities of daily living (ADLs); they become more than the task of getting a resident dressed and groomed for the day; they become opportunities to "connect" in meaningful ways for both care partners and residents.

I did not realize how powerful a loving touch approach to care was until I started seeing with my own eyes the positive changes in residents' behaviors and verbal responses when team members took the time to be present for them. When team members slowed down as they provided care, stopped to visit with residents, and showed the love that they feel in their hearts, the miracles began (Simard, 2012a). Residents who had ceased speaking in sentences would spontaneously blurt out "I love you" or simply "thank you." Their smiles replaced tears or sad faces, and resistance to care disappeared (Simard, 2012b). And it was so simple; team members just slowed down and showed their love. The power of loving touch is the foundation for Namaste Care and becomes the thread that weaves the fabric of the day to create a cocoon of love for the residents we care for and care about.

And so the Namaste Care day begins for our Namaste Care residents with a gentle awakening to the day. When words fail, Namaste Carers find other creative ways to communicate. Sally Callahan (2005) wrote lovingly of communicating with her mother, even when dementia had taken all language away. She said, "Somehow, together, we learned the language of eye hugs and heartspeak; through eye hugs and heartspeak we found a spiritual connection." She further commented on the feeling that not only was her mother calmed by their spiritual connection, but she was calmed herself. So, with heartspeak and eye hugs, care partners help residents greet the day.

## BEGINNING THE NAMASTE CARE DAY

A typical day in a nursing facility starts with the morning shift of care partners assisting residents with morning care. For a resident with advanced dementia that may mean providing total care, helping with all aspects of ADLs, then transferring them to a wheelchair or lounge chair. Residents are then taken to the dining room, where they may also need to be fed. On a good day in the United States, when all scheduled staff show up for work, the typical care partner is assigned six to eight residents. When staffing is less than optimal, each care partner might have 10 or more residents. "Frantic" and "rushed" are how care partners often describe their mornings. They speak of feeling frustrated that no matter how fast they work, they never really have the time to get all their tasks done. It's certainly not surprising that the turnover of care partners is exceptionally high in the long-term care industry in all the countries where I have worked. I know from conversations with administrators and directors of nursing that Namaste Care has had a positive impact on care partner turnover. They feel that it is because Namaste Care is a team effort, the process is more important than the task, and everyone on the team knows it and supports each other. I have seen a nurse make a bed when she realized that the care partner assigned to that room was the Namaste Carer that day. You can imagine how that care partner felt supported by nursing rather than fearing that she would be chastised for not making the bed.

Imagine, for a moment, how residents with advanced dementia must feel when team members are in a hurry to get their morning tasks done. When they have no way of knowing that it is indeed time to rise and shine, the constant commotion from highly energized staff must be frightening. Residents don't know where they are and what is expected of them. They may also feel hunger, are usually wet, and have not quite adjusted their sleepy body rhythms to waking up. It is the responsibility of care partners to help residents greet the day feeling safe and in the hands of a friend.

In a Namaste Care neighborhood, the morning begins with music—a soft, gentle beginning to each day with the sound of beautiful music or chirping birds filling the air. The music is usually a classical piece, love songs from the 1940s, or nature sounds. Morning is a time of awakening, the beginning of a new day, and the music should reflect that feeling. Music influences everyone in the neighborhood. Team members seem to slow down and approach their work with a lighter heart as beautiful music drifts through the corridors. Even if the facility does not have a Namaste

Care neighborhood, care partners can carry a small CD player with lovely "wake up" music to their resident's bedside in the morning.

Care partners always knock on the resident's door and identify themselves before entering the room. "Good morning, Mr. Black. I'm Carol, and I will help you get ready for breakfast." This is a simple but courteous way for staff members to enter a resident's room. When the resident appears to have heard the greeting and is beginning to wake up, a light touch lets the resident know that someone is there. Carly Hellen (1997) speaks of caring touch. Touch is the primary way we communicate with people who have lost their ability to understand verbal messages. We touch "hello" to let residents know we are there, we gently move parts of their bodies to dress them, and together with the sound of our voices, our facial expressions, and eye contact, we make waking up and getting ready for the day a less frightening experience. A man in the early stages of Alzheimer's disease described his memory loss as always feeling as if he had just woken up in the middle of a movie and had no idea what has just occurred. However, with soft reassurances and a loving touch approach from care partners, residents in Namaste Care are not as frightened and feel supported and comfortable in their world.

I wear a $3 \times 2$ name tag with "Joyce" in large black letters. Residents have such difficulty reading the usual name tag that has the name of the facility, a team member's name and title, and often a company logo. My name tag decreases their anxiety, and many residents who have never met me will call out "Hi, Joyce" as I pass by. State regulations require names and titles on facility name tags, and companies like their names on them as well, so team members will wear both tags. I worked with a nursing facility in Vermont called Helen Porter and many of the residents called the team members, whether male or female, "Helen"!

Some residents like the drapes opened early in the morning, and others prefer dim light; care partners need to know their residents' preferences so that the day begins in a way that suits the resident. The television set is turned off because we have found that care partners tend to talk less to the resident when the television is on. A person with advanced dementia is not usually aware enough to understand television programming, and news programs are filled with the bad news of the day. For too long, having the television on has been an excuse for not offering other programming. The television is definitely not a meaningful activity for residents with advanced dementia. Talking to a resident, even if it is one-sided, is a meaningful activity.

Care partners explain to the resident what is going to happen next and how he or she can help. For instance, a care partner might say, "Mr. Black, I'm going to help you get out of these wet clothes. I think you'll feel so much better. Can you help me by turning over?" Throughout morning care rituals, such as brushing teeth, washing faces, and combing hair, the care partners should urge residents to participate, even if it is just by opening their mouths or holding the face cloth, and then thank them for their help. Most people with dementia have some depression and I believe one of the causes is low self-esteem. Thanking a resident for whatever he or she can do reminds the person that he or she is still able to do for others.

Care partners praise residents' efforts to take part in their personal care. The intentional shift in terminology from *caregiver* to *care partner* reflects the need for the person on the receiving end of care to remain as independent as possible. Residents, even those with severe cognitive and physical impairments, must be given the opportunity to participate in their care. The care partner speaks in a low tone of voice and gives explicit step-by-step directions throughout the care process, saying, for instance, "John, I'm going to help you get dressed for breakfast. If you just give me a hug, I'll help you sit up," then, "Thanks for the hug," then "Now we will take off your gown; just lean forward like this" (models leaning forward). This is just one example of a positive way to involve the resident in his or her own care. Most residents in Namaste Care have lost the ability to communicate verbally, so care partners should watch for their nonverbal signs. The resident may communicate with facial expressions, body language, and sounds. If a resident is unable to make recognizable choices, the Namaste Carer continues to talk to the person, saying, for example, how handsome the resident will look in his clean shirt or that a woman has very beautiful hair that shines when it is combed. A resident who resists dressing and becomes agitated is perhaps communicating a wish to be left alone. In this case, care partners should respect them by providing as little care as possible, simply ensuring that the resident is clean and dry. Choice and control are always a part of Namaste Care.

People with dementia have difficulty dealing with the world around them, so eliminating "excess disabilities" is very important. This includes making sure that hearing aids are working properly, eyeglasses are clean, lighting is strong enough for them to see, and dentures fit. Unless the resident is clearly uncomfortable with wearing glasses, dentures, or hearing aids, these items should be maintained in good working order.

As the morning care ritual unfolds, care partners continually assess residents for signs of pain. Pain assessment begins the moment a care partner walks into the room and continues with every interaction. Care partners learn to read body language by watching the residents' body movements and facial expressions and listening to the tone of their voices (see Appendix F). If a care partner believes that a resident is experiencing pain or discomfort, he or she should report this to the nurse on the neighborhood.

Often, resisting morning care can indicate physical or mental distress. Taking time to sit with and talk to the resident is time consuming for care partners but a necessary part of Namaste Care. It is also important for care partners to know each resident's life story so that their conversations include important people and events in the residents' lives. Care partners find incredibly creative ways to work with residents. Successful ones know how to be creative and flexible.

## MOLLY

Molly was a difficult resident for the day staff, as she resisted most attempts to get her up and dressed peacefully. Molly had severe cognitive and physical impairments; in fact, Molly needed assistance with all personal care. In the morning, she was usually curled up in a tight ball of resistance and soaking wet. It was frustrating to care for her because she greeted all requests to cooperate with personal care by striking out and screaming at the care partners. She may have been frail and tiny, but she had a voice and strength that belied her size. No one wanted her on their assignment list, except for one care partner who was very successful in getting Molly up and dressed. She even coaxed smiles out of her.

The staff was desperate and called me for a consultation. A brief meeting, which I call a huddle, was scheduled to brainstorm approaches that might work with Molly. When the one care partner said she had no problems with Molly, we all stared at her. What, we asked, was her secret? She very hesitantly told us that when she entered Molly's room, she knocked on the door, said "Good morning, Grandma," and kissed Molly on the cheek. The care partner had stumbled on calling Molly "Grandma" when she had told Molly one day that she reminded her of her own grandma. Molly had smiled, and her eyes had lit up. This "Good morning, Grandma" greeting became part of their special relationship. After Molly was awake, the care partner would say that she was taking Fluffy (the cat who had been Molly's best friend for years) off the bed so she could eat her cat food. She pantomimed removing the cat from the bed, after which Molly was happy to cooperate with her morning care.

How did the care partner know about Fluffy, we asked? She replied that she had been as frustrated as the rest of her teammates, so when she saw family and friends visiting, she made it a point to find out all she could about Molly. They told her about Fluffy and the strong relationship between Molly and her cat. Molly's daughter remarked that her mother was very protective of her cat and had slept with Fluffy for years. It occurred to the assistant that Molly might be curled into a ball to cuddle the cat. In spite of her advanced dementia, Molly had a strong connection with memories of the cat. Once the cat was out of bed and happy, Molly was content to allow her "granddaughter" to help her get ready for the day.

Creatively finding approaches that work makes job responsibilities fun and less like work. It has been suggested that a new beatitude for nursing facility staff might look like this:

Blessed are the care partners
Who are flexible
For they shall not break!

## PREPARING THE NAMASTE CARE ROOM

Once breakfast has been served and the majority of residents are fed and groomed, the Namaste Care room is prepared for the morning activities. The daily program usually begins around 9:30 A.M., but this depends on the facility's breakfast schedule. Responsibility for preparing the Namaste Care room for the morning program depends on how the program is staffed.

These are some of the creative ways nursing facilities prepare the room for programming:

- If there is a separate position for a Namaste Carer, that person may help with breakfast because so many residents need assistance with meals. Then he or she gathers the morning supplies and prepares the room.

- When one of the neighborhood care partners is chosen to be the Namaste Carer, he or she alerts other team members to watch the residents assigned to them while they are preparing the room.

- If the room has been used for dining, the housekeeping staff cleans the floor. In some communities, the activity staff will help to get the room set up for the daily programming.

See box 5.1 for a list of the tasks to be completed in preparing the room for the Namaste Care program. All supplies must be in the room before the programming begins so that the Namaste Carer does not have to leave the room once the program begins. For the safety of residents, the room is never to be left unattended when residents are present.

These are just recommendations based on my experience; however, each facility should develop its own list of tasks. It is useful to post this list at the nursing station because occasionally someone who usually does not work in the Namaste Care room will be asked to take over the program for the day. A list of residents participating in the Namaste Care program should also be posted at all nurses' stations, in the wellness areas in assisted living, and in the assignment books so that all team members know which residents attend Namaste Care. Special diets that include instructions for residents who have swallowing difficulties should be noted with each resident's name.

## OPENING THE NAMASTE CARE ROOM

The team member responsible for opening the Namaste Care Room will complete the following tasks prior to beginning the daily programming:

- Gather beverages for the day: juice, water, supplements, ingredients for "smoothies," and so forth. Whenever possible, pour each resident a beverage in a cup or glass with the resident's name. This will save time and have beverages available as soon as the residents enter the room and have been made comfortable.

- Gather food items for the day: oranges, pineapple, ice cream, puddings, cookies, lollipops, and so forth. Try to avoid using supplements, because they are expensive, and residents seem to prefer food items that are what they have enjoyed in the past. Ideally, Namaste Care rooms have refrigerators so that food and beverages can be stored safely. Someone must be responsible for regularly cleaning out the refrigerator. In some facilities, this is done by the dietary department. In other facilities, the Namaste Carer is responsible for cleaning and maintaining the refrigerator according to regulations. State and federal regulations require a temperature chart to be filled in each day by a team member.

- Make sure food supplies are available, such as napkins, a plastic serrated knife for cutting oranges, spoons and straws, and so forth.

- Ensure that all food and beverage products are labeled with the date the programming is taking place.

- Ensure that any exposed food is in a closed container or place wrapping on the exposed food along with the date the programming is taking place.

- Remove any out-of-date food and beverage products from the refrigerator.

- Survey the room for cleanliness.

- Gather towels, face cloths, basins, soap, lotion, mouth swabs, shaving cream, safety razors, and other items needed for the morning programming and personal care.

- Make sure pillowcases, quilts, and blankets are available and are clean.

- Spend some time making the room look as homey as possible with tablecloths, fresh flowers, and items that will help to make the room look like a living room.

*(Box continued on next page)*

**OPENING THE NAMASTE CARE ROOM** *(Continued)*

- Spray the room with lavender or turn on the aroma diffuser.
- Water plants.
- Set the heat or air conditioning to a comfortable setting for the residents.
- Turn on the music.
- Play an appropriate DVD.
- Inform team members that the Namaste Care Room is opened.
- Hang a sign on the door that welcomes people into the Namaste Care room.

## CREATING THE APPROPRIATE AMBIENCE IN THE NAMASTE CARE ROOM

When residents enter the Namaste Care room, they should feel as if they are enveloped in a calm, soothing environment, like being wrapped in a cocoon. Creating the ambience for the daily program includes playing appropriate music, infusing the room with a soothing scent, and setting the lights to help create a soft and pleasant aura. These three elements are to be in place before residents are taken into the room.

### Music

As anyone in the caregiving profession knows, music is a universal language. There is some evidence that even comatose patients respond to music. The area of the brain that responds to music is the last to be affected by Alzheimer's disease (Cuddy & Duffin, 2005). Music helps create the calming, enveloping mood that permeates the Namaste Care room. Consider the following types of music to convey different kinds of moods:

- New Age music that is soft and soothing for quiet time

- Nature sounds—birds singing, waterfalls trickling, and the echo of animals in the wild—for stimulating the senses during an activity
- Big-band sounds for range-of-motion exercises or to help awaken residents before lunch and dinner
- Broadway musicals such as *Oklahoma, The Sound of Music,* or *The King and I* may get a reaction and have residents clapping or tapping their toes in time to the music
- Love songs from Bing Crosby, Frank Sinatra, and Patti Page for the afternoon when spouses visit
- Classical music; Pachelbel's Canon is a popular piece for creating a restful feeling
- Cultural music, depending on the background of the residents, such as Mexican mariachi, Czech polkas, folk songs from European countries, or calypso and reggae music from Latin American countries
- Religious music such as hymns for Sunday or Jewish songs for the Friday and Saturday Sabbath

Part of the adventure of Namaste Care is trying different music to create the mood that is consistent with what is occurring in the room, what meaningful activity is taking place. For instance, as the residents come into the room, the mood is tranquil on most days. Perhaps after a particularly dreary and rainy few days, everyone's mood needs to be lifted, and "Oh, What a Beautiful Morning" greets team members and residents. Before lunch and dinner, sounds from the big-band era help wake residents up for the meal. In Australia, "Waltzing Matilda" is a happy way to wake up residents. On Sunday hymns might help residents recognize the Sabbath day. And of course we always strive for laughter as part of the day. One wonderful activity professional I worked with came into the room wearing a rainbow wig and clown red nose accompanied by circus music featuring a calliope! Selecting music is one of the creative ways each Namaste Carer can add his or her own individual touch to the day. If your facility has access to a music therapist, he or she can also be helpful in selecting music.

## Scents

Lavender is the preferred scent for the Namaste Care room. Studies have shown that this scent decreases anxiety and is a calming agent (Lin et al., 2007). The scent must be strong enough for anyone entering the room to smell. A diffuser is the most effective way to fill the room with a fragrance. If the diffuser is electrical, it must be approved by the maintenance department. Other options for scenting the room include plug-ins, linen spray, and reed diffusers if placed out of residents' reach. In some cases a lavender room spray is used to make sure the room has the scent of lavender as soon as it opens because a diffuser may take some time to permeate the room. It also helps to have a stronger scent if the room is also used as a dining room and the smell of food has lingered after the meal. Lighted incense sticks are never used because of the fire hazard they create. I have heard some concern that surveyors do not like scent because they do not want it used as a cover-up for unpleasant odors. If questioned by a surveyor, explain why the scent is used and that it is part of the Namaste Care environment.

## Lighting

Lighting helps to set the mood of the room. Harsh overhead lighting can be avoided by asking the maintenance department to install dimming switches for ceiling lights. Natural lighting is always the best option, but some rooms do not have windows large enough to offer sufficient light. Floor lamps might be the answer because this type of lighting is softer and helps make the room look homey.

## GATHERING RESIDENTS

Gathering residents for the morning program is sometimes challenging for care partners because of the time it takes to get their morning assignments completed. Some facilities I work with assign one or two managers and other team members to help transport residents to the morning activities that include taking them to the Namaste Care room: culture change in action! Dedicating 15 minutes to helping care partners in the morning is not a problem for most team members and managers and helps the care partners feel supported—a real team.

## OPENING THE NAMASTE CARE ROOM

After supplies, beverages, and food items are gathered, music is playing, lights are dimmed, and the room is staged with tablecloths, flowers, and other items to make it look and feel warm and inviting, the door is opened and the Namaste Care program begins. It's always interesting to see the reaction of the residents to the sensory impact of entering the room even when they have just been in the same room for breakfast. With the music, the scent of lavender, and the look of the room, it feels different for team members and residents. The room helps to show how unique this program is within the nursing facility. Families, staff, and residents become quieter and more respectful in this space, and everything slows down. One resident's spouse described entering the Namaste Care room as being "enveloped by a giant hug."

## WELCOME TO NAMASTE CARE

Each resident who enters the Namaste Care room is greeted by name and touched in some gentle and respectful manner. Welcoming them as a unique person is a way to honor the spirit within, the meaning of *Namaste*. Using a preferred name or title is one way to do this. For example, in one Namaste Care program, one of the residents is affectionately called "Gramps" and another, who had been a surgeon, is addressed as Doctor Smith.

All residents, family members, friends, and team members are made to feel welcomed in the Namaste Care room and encouraged to join the program. The door may be closed to keep the noise level down, but a sign on the door saying "Welcome to Namaste Care, please come in!" gives the appropriate message to visitors and team members. It is important to educate everyone so that they can come and go as necessary. For instance, if it is the residents' day for a shower, rather than leaving them in their rooms until the care partner has time to give the showers, the residents can be taken to the Namaste Care room in their robes and slippers so they will not be isolated. When the care partners have time to give the residents their showers, they come into the room, tell the residents that they will be leaving for a little while, and say goodbye to the Namaste Carer. When the showers have been completed, the residents are returned to the Namaste Care room and again greeted by the Namaste Carer.

I prefer to have the door open just enough for the resident who wanders to feel as if he or she can enter the room. We have feedback from nursing that having Namaste Care lowers falls because the wandering resident finds the room and falls asleep. It has also been interesting for me to see residents in the early stage of dementia who choose not to attend regular activity programs but who come to Namaste Care. This is especially true for residents in assisted living communities. I think the calm environment draws them in, and they are not overstimulated by an activity program.

Sometimes medications are dispensed while residents are in Namaste Care, but treatments are not. Residents are taken from the room for anything that may be an infringement on their privacy. Families also should know that they can come into the room at any time and either take their loved one out or sit next to them and be part of the program.

## GETTING COMFORTABLE

All residents who enter the Namaste Care room should be placed in a comfortable chair. They may be transferred from a wheelchair and placed in a lounge chair or simply made more comfortable in whatever chair they normally use. Two care partners are needed for transferring a resident from a wheelchair to a lounge chair for safety reasons. To make sure residents are positioned correctly, it is a good idea to ask a physical therapist to look at how residents are seated at least once a month. This is especially important for residents who have contractures or are at high risk for skin breakdown.

Correct positioning in an appropriate chair will help decrease these potential skin problems. At this stage of their disease, they sleep quite a bit, so a reclining lounge chair is more comfortable than a wheelchair. If a resident is receiving hospice care in the United States, the hospice organization may supply a lounge chair or reclining wheelchair for their patient as part of the requirements to provide medical equipment related to their disease.

In recent years residents have become more and more disabled, and a lifting device is needed so that they can be moved from a wheelchair to a lounge chair. The main problem with this is that it takes two staff members for the transfer, and care must be taken to prevent skin tears. In the United Kingdom, care homes are not responsible for providing lounge chairs, and if families cannot afford to purchase them, residents are in wheelchairs or are "bedbound," a word I would like to see disappear from our vocabulary. Some care homes are getting creative, having fundraisers to purchase chairs, asking families to donate chairs after a resident has died, placing footstools in front of the facility's living room chairs, and using pillows and blankets to help position residents more comfortably. When the residents are comfortably seated, their shoes are removed and tucked under the chair, and belts and bras are loosened.

A quilt or some other covering is then tucked around the resident because this seems to help them to feel secure and warm. Several years ago at a conference I attended, a nurse presented a poster session on decreasing agitation among people with dementia by tucking bed sheets around them at night; the same idea has been applied here. Also, as people age, their metabolism changes, and many residents are cold even in warm weather. It can be difficult for care partners, who are racing around the neighborhood caring for their residents in the heat of summer, to understand how cold residents may be, but it is an important point to reinforce. A variety of coverings can be used; twin-sized quilts are the most popular because they are easy to wash, do not need to be ironed, and are comfortable and cozy. Washable afghans and twin-size blankets are also good choices. Twin sheets can be used during warm weather or for residents who prefer a light covering. All coverings should be colorful, not institutional white. Colorful prints and soft colors create a warm look and help the Namaste Care room look more like a family room.

Each resident needs his or her own blanket, quilt, or sheet for infection control compliance. They must be kept clean and stored in the Namaste Care room to control how many times they are washed so that they remain as soft and fluffy as possible. Often they are placed in a large zippered garment bag with the resident's name on it or a large zip-locked bag and hung on a rod in the closet or storage cabinet. If the room can be secured and there is enough space, attractive storage containers can be used. When a resident has a special stuffed animal, neck pillow, or other personal item, they can also be placed in the bag or storage container. Every item used by residents must be labeled to meet infection control standards. We do not use a laundry pen to mark blankets because it is permanent, and we reuse blankets and quilts after a resident has died.

## SEATING ARRANGEMENTS

Where each resident is placed in the room depends on the needs and interests of the resident and the size of the room. Some residents enjoy being grouped together so they feel the presence of each other. Other residents enjoy being close to a window to feel the sunlight or to watch the colors and the movement of the birds. Sometimes placement is a matter of practicality. For instance, when it is Mrs. Gold's day for a bath, she is placed near the door so that she can be taken from the room without disrupting other residents. I have fond memories of Charlie, who loved hiking in the mountains of Vermont. His chair always faced the window, where he could see them. We honored his past love of hiking in this small way. If the room has a television, a nature DVD may be playing, and some residents might be grouped around it. Try to avoid placing residents in a circle around the room; it looks institutional and not very inviting. As soon as they are seated, a beverage is offered.

## ACTIVITIES OF DAILY LIVING AS MEANINGFUL ACTIVITIES

Each Namaste Care resident has a small zippered bag with his or her own personal care supplies: a comb or brush, emery board, nail clippers, and personal items such as a favorite scent or lipstick. One resident's family wanted their mother to wear a gold cross necklace she was never without before she moved to a nursing facility. They were afraid that it would get lost, and so the family kept it at home and put it on their mother when visiting. The Namaste Carer offered to keep the cross in her zippered bag and put it on their mother every day while she was in the Namaste Care room. The Namaste Carer did advise the family that this was not a foolproof solution, but it lowered the chances of the cross disappearing. The family accepted the offer and was very comforted when they saw their mother caressing the cross, even when she appeared to be sleeping. Rather than storing these bags in an unattractive plastic container, I often place them in a decorative basket. Little touches like this make the program less institutional and can help change the look of a room. Park Avenue Care Center in London uses small cosmetic bags that are colorful and washable, with flowered patterns for the women and bold stripes for the men. The bags are placed on small tables that seem to be a favorite of care homes in the United Kingdom. In this care home, the table also might have a picture of the resident's family or some personal item, such as a small soccer ball that was on the table of one of the men. On the day I visited each table also had a small vase with a fresh tulip. The tables are somewhat like the over-bed tables used in hospitals and nursing homes, but they did not look as institutional and were very practical. I can also see using "TV tables," also called tray tables or snack tables. These tables are quite inexpensive and would be functional yet attractive when placed next to a resident in the Namaste Care room.

## MEANINGFUL ACTIVITIES
## AND THE POWER OF LOVING TOUCH

### Moisturizing the Face

When the majority of residents are in the Namaste Care room, programming begins. Skin becomes drier with age, and applying cold cream or moisturizer to residents' faces after they are washed is a wonderful reminiscence activity. In particular, Pond's Cold Cream has an aroma that women appear to remember. If each resident does not have his or her own face cream; one large jar is available. The Namaste Carer uses a plastic spoon or cotton bud and medication dispensing cups. The amount of cream needed for each woman is put into the cup and the spoon or cotton bud placed in the trash container after use. This avoids any danger of cross-contamination. At the start of each day, every woman in the Namaste Care room should have her face washed with a wet, warm cloth (but not dried, in order to keep moisture on the skin) and face cream applied. Namaste Carers do not use gloves unless necessary because the power of loving touch is more effective skin to skin.

I never thought about using face cream on men until I began working with Arden Courts. They purchased Ponds for everyone in the program, including men. I was surprised to see how many men enjoyed having their faces caressed with this softly scented cream. I now suggest adding a drop of "Old Spice" aftershave to face cream is a lovely way to add reminiscence to this activity.

## Shaving

Although most grooming is usually completed before a resident is taken to the Namaste Care room, shaving men in the Namaste Care room can turn a basic ADL into a pleasurable activity and create an incredible sensory opportunity. Shaving must be done by a trained care partner or nurse according to regulations. The act of shaving in public could be viewed as a violation of privacy, so be sensitive. If the resident enjoys a special shave in the Namaste Care room, make sure it is noted in his care plan. Make this grooming task an enjoyable process by shaving the way men were shaved years ago. As you do, the scent of shaving cream will permeate the Namaste Care room, a welcome reminder of days gone by. When a resident resists the process of shaving, discontinue the activity immediately.

### EARL

Earl was the lead care partner on the Namaste Care wing. On most days, he was responsible for shaving Jerry, one particular resident who did not like to be shaved. Earl was a good care partner and used all the correct approaches. The end result was that some days Jerry was not shaved and sprouted bristles that look great on Tom Cruise but were upsetting to the resident's family. Other days, Earl won by successfully dodging the resident's attempts to hit him. One day, Earl took Jerry to the Namaste Care room to give him an old-fashioned shave. The Namaste Carer gave Earl the barber cape, safety razors, shaving cream, and Old Spice aftershave lotion. He was pleasantly surprised to find that Jerry actually smiled when he was shaved. Of course, that might have been because he remembered that when he was younger, going to a barber for a shave was a luxury and a pleasurable experience. The cape and supplies gave him clues, so he did not resist shaving because he knew what was going to occur. Maybe he also remembered that when the shave ended he would get a kiss on the cheek from the Namaste Carer, who declared him the handsomest man in the room!

Although shaving is primarily a male necessity, facial hair on women also needs attention. Removing facial hair on women should be done in the privacy of their rooms or behind a screen in the Namaste Care room. Using a safety razor (which must be disposed of afterward), facial hair can usually be removed quickly and without any problems. Taking pride in how each resident looks shows respect for the residents and their families. One Namaste Carer removes facial hair from a woman when everyone has left the room for lunch, so it is done as an individual activity and in privacy. Families are often embarrassed by the facial hair on their mother but do not know what to do about it because electrolysis is not a good option for women with advanced dementia. They are grateful that this is done for their mothers who were very well groomed when they were younger.

### Make-Up

Applying make-up, such as light lipstick, may be a welcome activity; however, more extensive make-up might be appropriate for residents who have been accustomed to wearing full make-up every day, like Eleanor.

## *ELEANOR*

Eleanor was a model years ago. The family proudly showed pictures of her modeling the latest Paris fashions. Even when she was older, she loved dressing up and would never think about going out without full make-up. Actually, family members noticed the beginning of dementia when she started looking, in their words, bizarre. Eyebrow liner went every which way, far above or below eyebrows, and eye shadow was much too dark. Lipstick went beyond the lips, and her hair, once meticulously colored and maintained with a weekly trip to the beauty parlor, was uncombed on most days. It was apparent that Eleanor was forgetting beauty shop appointments, something she never would have done before. As the disease progressed, she lost all ability to groom herself and did not seem to care anymore. It was devastating to the family to see their mother looking like this. Namaste Care recognized that the best way to honor Eleanor was to make time for special grooming and for dressing her in the beautiful clothing provided by the family. Eleanor once again regained the title of beauty queen.

## Hair Care

Most women and some men enjoy having their hair combed. In the advanced stage of dementia, beauty shop appointments are often dismissed as unnecessary and can even cause discomfort for the resident. We know that residents possess inner beauty, but it is also important to maintain their exterior beauty. Short hair is easier to groom; if a woman can tolerate it, consider permanents and hair coloring if that is her family's preference. One pleasing activity in the morning is to comb everyone's hair with gentle strokes. Most residents enjoy the attention. It is important to keep hair care items clearly labeled and separated for hygiene reasons.

## *DORIS*

My own mother always told me that no matter what physical condition she was in, she wanted to be a "natural blonde" until the day she died. She had a very disabling stroke that left her unable to speak, but she had her hair colored while she was in the nursing home. As an only child, I was responsible for making sure that no one would be looking at her in the casket and see gray roots! At age 87, Doris was a "natural blonde" for her funeral. I'm sure no one suspected she colored her hair.

## SARA

When I was visiting the first Namaste Care program in Bennington, Vermont, I observed Sara, a care partner, lovingly braiding the long hair of Ann, a resident who seemed to have progressed in her dementia to the point of almost never responding to any kind of touch. When asked why she bothered to take time to do this when Ann did not seem to care whether her hair was braided or not, Sara responded that she had seen a picture of Ann in her younger days and noticed how beautifully her hair was braided. Because she found so little she could do that would be special just for Ann, this became her way of showing respect and honor for this resident's natural beauty.

## Nail and Hand Care

One day per week, Namaste Care can schedule a Beauty Day to simulate the services of a beauty shop. Some facilities have a Spa Day where they do nails, soak feet, and provide back rubs. An activity team member can assist with soaking, cleaning, and filing fingernails (nail cutting must be done by a care partner or nurse). It is easier to keep fingernails short and clean. A light nail polish can be used if the resident previously used nail polish, or simply buff nails to keep them shiny and healthy. These days are a special activity for residents in Namaste Care.

## Hand Washing and Massage

All residents in Namaste Care have their hands washed and massaged in warm water. When the room has a sink, individual basins are filled with warm, soapy water and one hand at a time is placed in the water as the Namaste Carer talks to the resident. If no sink is available, the wet warm washcloths are kept in a plastic bag. Residents' hands are then dried, and lotion is massaged on the hands and arms.

## MICHELE

Michele was the director of nursing in one of the facilities with a Namaste Care program. Her support was invaluable to implementing Namaste Care. One day when Michele came into the Namaste Care room, she noticed a resident with an anxious expression on her face and clenched fists. The Namaste Carer who was responsible for the program that day told Michele that in spite of all she had tried with this resident, there was no getting her to relax so her hands could be washed.

Michele went into action. She took a basin of warm water and sat next to the resident. She spoke very softly to the woman, and the resident gradually allowed her hands to be placed in the basin. Slowly, the woman opened her clenched fists, and her face showed pleasure, all traces of anxiety gone. Michele took the face cloth, filled it with water, and wrung it out, making a small waterfall. At this, the resident broke into the most joyful smile and exclaimed, "This is wonderful!" One seemingly small moment, but that is what Namaste Care is all about, one human touching another.

## REALISTIC STUFFED ANIMALS AND DOLLS

Part of getting to know residents is discovering whether realistic stuffed animals or lifelike dolls will bring additional comfort to their lives. I have seen residents who have stopped talking to people talk to babies or dogs. Most residents have had a pet sometime in their lives, so lifelike animals may remind them of their furry friends. If a resident does not like animals, he or she will let you know. Men seem to be soothed by and enjoy large dogs that are easier to hold. Women like cats and soft rabbits. They must be as lifelike as possible, no elephants or teddy bears, and they must be assigned to one resident for infection control purposes and cleaned as needed. Often they are stored with the blanket or quilt in a large storage bag.

I resisted giving women dolls for years, until I saw a woman who had been depressed for as long as I had known her smile and love her "baby." She talked to the baby, showed the baby to everyone who came into the room, and slept with the baby snuggled in her arms. The most dramatic story I have ever heard about using realistic dolls to improve quality of life happened in the United Kingdom.

## ABIGAIL

Abigail was a resident who had never married and had no children. She often wandered around the neighborhood, seemingly looking for something or, as it turned out, someone. One day Abigail wandered into the living room and spied a realistic doll. She took the baby in her arms and said, "At last I found you. I will never let you go again." Abigail stopped wandering and became a loving mother who enjoyed sitting in the Namaste Care room with her "baby." One day a care partner came into her room and saw that Abigail had her nightgown pulled down and appeared to be "nursing" the baby. The care partner quietly left the room, respecting her privacy. The charge nurse thought that perhaps Abigail had been forced to surrender her baby when she was a young, unmarried girl, something that would have been fairly common years ago. If indeed that had happened to her, she may have been feeling guilty about giving up her baby her entire life. Now that she had "found" her baby and could care for it, she seemed to have finally found peace in her life as she lovingly cared for her child, proudly showing her to everyone.

I am now a believer in using realistic dolls and stuffed animals that look real when no other item provides the comfort they do; whatever works works! Families and visitors must be told about the comforting effects of these pets and babies because we do not want them to think that Namaste Care infantilizes any resident.

## ANDREW

Andrew was a resident in a care home near Sydney, Australia. When I met him he had a child's wall hanging on his lap. It was made of burlap and featured a large lion's head with a mane of long red yarn. Andrew was fiddling with the mane, twisting and turning the yarn. I asked why they were using this children's accessory, and the Namaste Carer responded that Andrew had been a telephone technician, and he seemed to be trying to fix telephone lines. I found the maintenance worker and asked him whether he had a telephone that was broken that I could use. When he brought me one, I asked him to request Andrew's help in "fixing" it. With a smile on his face, Andrew took the phone and immediately began to "work" on it. I quietly took the lion away, and Andrew had an adult item that gave him pleasure. One day as I was leaving the room I saw that Andrew was "fixing" several tele-phones that were on a table in front of him. I thanked him for his help, and he replied, "Don't you have any phones that work in this place?"

This is just one example of knowing the resident's life history (Appendix E) and finding a way to use adult items to engage him or her.

## MORNING NOURISHMENTS

Never underestimate the power of food. It represents care, po-liteness, giving, and receiving. Families focus on food. Can you remember when you were small and not feeling well, your worried mother hovering around the bed trying to tempt you with food? She was so grateful when you would eat or drink something. Offer-ing food and beverages as a social ritual is ingrained into our very being. We greet people in our homes with an offer of food or drink. Socialization usually involves food and beverages.

As residents' cognitive impairments increase, their appetites decrease, and eating problems arise (Gillick & Mitchell, 2002). It is part of the natural progression of the disease. Weight loss and dehydration are almost always concerns in the advanced stage of the disease. The ability to feel hunger and thirst seems to disappear in advanced dementia. Although this is a normal, natural way for the body to prepare for this last part of its life journey, it is very troubling for families, may lead to dehydration, and increases the risk of infections.

Each resident is unique, so rather than just accepting food re-fusal as normal for advanced dementia, it is good practice to assess any resident who begins resisting food for apathy and depression. Antidepressants and other medications may help to improve mood and appetite but may cause some burden to the resident. Medica-tions may produce a dry mouth, constipation or diarrhea, and a range of other unpleasant symptoms. In Namaste Care, an effort is made to tempt residents with small offerings of sweet and easy-to-swallow food and beverages. The atmosphere in the Namaste Care room seems to stimulate appetites; perhaps it's having others around them. Or maybe the individual attention they receive stimulates their appetite. I have found that until residents begin to actively die, they seem to enjoy drinking and eating while they are in the Namaste Care room. When I first started working with activity professionals, they would often come back from lunch at a restaurant with residents who needed help eating while in the nursing home. They would tell me that when these same residents were in the restaurant, they suddenly became very independent with eating skills, more social, and very polite. Their long-term memory surfaced, and they knew how to act while in a restaurant. Perhaps the same logic could be applied in the Namaste Care room with residents who have advanced dementia. Their long-term memory of how to act in a room that feels as if they are in someone's home kicks in, and they remember to at least try to eat and drink what is offered.

## Swallowing Problems

Occasionally, a resident will have problems with swallowing as the disease reaches its final stage. Namaste Care team members should watch for any swallowing problems. Observation is critical when residents have limited means to communicate verbally. When swallowing difficulties occur, it may be helpful to have a speech therapist, one who understands the Namaste Care concept of quality of life, evaluate the resident. Sometimes, a feeding tube is considered. For residents with advanced dementia, however, feeding tubes do not extend life and have many drawbacks. For more information on feeding tubes, see Chapter 8.

Registered dietitians, who are skilled in providing nutritional assessments, can recommend different textures of food or show how to thicken liquids. However, thickening liquids may not prevent aspiration and may make swallowing more difficult and lead to dehydration (Campbell-Taylor, 2008). For safety reasons, Namaste Care team members should be informed about any residents who have swallowing difficulties. Residents who have swallowing difficulties, or who pouch food in their cheeks, should sit upright as they are being fed to aid in the swallowing process.

## Beverages

In Namaste Care, food and liquids are offered continually by hand as a normal part of the day, as opposed to usual practice of passing out beverages in the morning and afternoon. Residents are offered a beverage in a cup marked with her or his name as soon as they are made comfortable in the room. Then when the Namaste Carer has finished washing a resident's face and hands, applying moisturizer, and combing his or her hair, the resident is offered more to drink. Then the Namaste Carer does the morning routine with another resident, offers him or her a beverage, then returns to the first resident and offers more sips. Many times other care partners and managers will come in the Namaste Care room just to assist with continuous beverage service. This occurs in the morning and afternoon sessions. Nurses have reported to me that increasing the amount of liquid consumed by residents in the Namaste Care program decreases infections, especially urinary tract infections and skin tears.

We offer residents a variety of juices, so they always have a choice. Cranberry juice is especially beneficial for preventing urinary tract infections in women. Milk and buttermilk add calories but are constipating. Ginger ale seems to be favored as a comfort drink. The sweetness is appealing, but the bubbles may be bothersome; leaving the bottle uncapped will decrease the number of bubbles but keep the taste intact. Beverages are served at room temperature rather than cold or with ice. In the summer and for some residents, cold drinks are preferred. Using a flexible straw will reduce the shock of the cold liquid. I like to use straws because I believe one of the last reflexes to disappear at the end of life is one of the first we recognize in healthy newborns: the ability to suck. Straws, especially short ones, do not require much energy for sucking and seem to be effective even for residents who usually do not drink (Asplund, Norberg, & Adolfsson, 1991; Franssen, Reisberg, Kluger, Sinaiko, & Boja, 1991). Sometimes before giving them the straw, I put some of the liquid on their lips to give them a taste of what will be offered. We always give a choice of at least two beverages. Sometimes even the usually nonverbal resident will be able to choose a beverage. However, food or liquid is never forced on a resident; we honor their choices, difficult as it is for Namaste Carers and for families.

In Australia the care homes use sipping cups that have been marked with the resident's name and are washed in the facility dishwasher. Some have two handles, which seems to help residents hold the cups and drink independently without spilling the contents. Another facility uses colorful travel mugs because they look like something anyone would use. Most facilities use plastic throwaway cups with covers and a straw. The cup is marked with the resident's name and kept nearby so that anyone can easily find the resident's beverage and offer it to her or him. Continuous hydration is an important part of the Namaste Care program. Families like hearing that their loved one enjoyed some nourishment that day. Even better, ask families to offer refreshments during their visits if allowed by regulations.

Families often welcome the chance to do something productive, such as helping their loved ones to eat and drink. This meaningful activity can ease the difficulty and frustration of visits with a family member who is no longer able to communicate. Families and Namaste Care team members always offer food in a way that is gentle, kind, and respectful. Even if the resident does not seem to understand, he or she is told that a delicious drink has been prepared. Namaste Carers place the resident's hands around the cup and encourage every sip that is taken. If it is difficult to rouse a resident, gently stroke his or her cheek while talking about drinking something. This gesture may stimulate the resident into taking nourishment.

## Fruit

Fruits are a wonderful source of nourishment and hydration for residents with advanced dementia. Pineapple is appealing to some residents; it smells good and tastes good. Canned, crushed pineapple is easy to swallow, stimulates the saliva and digestive juices, and has a chemical effect on the mouth that aids good mouth hygiene. Oranges sliced in quarters are also enjoyed by many residents.

First, hold the orange slice close to tempt the resident with the fruit's smell, then dribble a few drops on the person's lips, which can stimulate him or her to suck on the orange slice. Witness the pure delight!

### SAM

> Sam was a wisp of a man who hardly ate or drank. The director of nursing once remarked that she thought Sam was alive only because of the love surrounding him in Namaste Care. Care partners were so tender as they moved him from the chair to bed. It was as if they held a tiny sparrow in their hands. He had gentle but very aware eyes and almost no recognizable speech. Somehow it still seemed that he knew you were present for him. One day, I decided to give Sam a taste of orange. I approached him with a piece of orange and introduced myself. When the orange piece was near his nose, Sam immediately opened his eyes, and the eyes said "Yes!" I gave him a slice, and he sucked on the orange with such vigor that his strength surprised me. Then, he looked at me with such gratefulness and love that I was hooked. From that moment on, my visits to the facility always included Sam and an orange slice. I know it was special for him and provided moments for me that will forever remain in my mind.

## Lollipops

Lollipops are a fun way to keep mouths moist. Most residents will not chew on them because they lack the teeth or the strength to bite down. As always, assessment and observation are important to prevent problems. Residents usually respond positively when a Namaste Carer says he or she has a lollipop for them. Their smiles brighten the room. Small lollipops are inexpensive and easy to suck. Family members usually smile too when they come into the Namaste Care room and find their loved one sucking on a lollipop.

## Smoothies

Namaste Care rooms should have blenders to make smoothies. These mixtures of fruit and high-calorie liquid are easy to make and are beneficial for the resident who has not eaten breakfast or who needs the extra calories. These delicious nourishments can be made at a moment's notice and in small amounts. Use high-calorie products such as ice cream, sherbets, and canned fruit that satisfy the sweet tooth and may help decrease weight loss.

## Yogurt

Yogurt is a natural food that is easily swallowed and comes in a variety of flavors. Yogurt carries less danger of choking and aspirating than milk for residents who have difficulty swallowing. It also improves the microbes in the intestines. Yogurt can be purchased in small, individual servings, and many include sweet fruit syrup.

## BRINGING THE MORNING TO A CLOSE

About 20 minutes before care partners begin to take their residents out of the Namaste Care room and prepare them for lunch, the lights are turned up and livelier music is played. This is to help wake up residents who are sleeping and stimulate them to be ready for their meal. This is a time to have some fun and provide clues as to the season or an upcoming holiday. Providing a scent to harmonize with the weather and the season is a good way to accomplish this. Many stores provide a variety of essential oils, which are expensive, or candles or sachets, which are quite inexpensive. If scented candles are used, the wicks need to be removed so they cannot be lit. Although lavender is the preferred scent to start the Namaste Care day, the Namaste Carer must use good judgment and creativity to try different scents to coordinate with the meaningful activity that is occurring or to reflect the season. The lavender scent is used to help residents feel as if they are entering a calm, peaceful environment. The scent used before their meal has another purpose, and that is to stimulate them.

Scents can be very effective when coordinated with music and reminiscence items. For instance, the facilities I work with near the ocean on Cape Cod, Massachusetts, use the scent of the sea and play the song "Old Cape Cod" that was popular in the 1950s. Some days residents wear sun hats and basins of beach sand are available for them to feel and there is a DVD of squawking seagulls flying over the ocean. These sensory items may reach long-ago memories of happy days on vacation at the beach.

During the winter the scent of cinnamon provides a warm feeling while Bing Crosby sings "Let It Snow" and a basin of snow is passed around for residents to touch. Spring scents include flowers such as lily-of-the-valley, lilacs, and hyacinths. I love when team members bring in fresh flowers, and in the spring they seem to bloom everywhere and of course are free. Even the lowly dandelion can evoke a smile from residents. Once we had a room full of residents blowing the seed head (I had to look this up because I had no idea what to call the flower after it stopped blooming) off in every direction. The mess created by this exercise was not appreciated by the housekeeper, but the residents loved it.

Summer brings the smell of fragrant roses, watermelon, and rain, with colorful umbrellas for residents to hold. A gentle spray of water helps them feel the rain. During the crisp fall weather, the aroma of apples and cinnamon is appropriate. You may have some more alert residents who can make clove oranges to put in the room. So far, the smell of burning leaves has not been bottled, but perhaps someone will figure out how to produce that familiar scent. Long before regulations made it illegal to burn leaves in your backyard, this activity was a family tradition and a strong indication that fall had arrived.

The best scents are the real things. One Namaste Carer kept the room filled with lilacs when they were in bloom. Another brought freshly cut grass during the summer that brought smiles from the women and looks from the men that seemed to say, "Oh no, the grass needs to be cut!" Supplies for programming are as basic as the program itself. It is all about the fundamentals of life, and nature is one of them. The smell of bread baking is another wonderful morning scent. Consider purchasing a bread maker and easy-to-use mixes; as an added bonus, the residents may be able to eat the homemade bread.

Keeping fresh flowers in the room is always a welcome touch. However, make sure that no residents are allergic to the flowers.

Consider purchasing African violets, which bloom year-round. Or talk to a local funeral home about delivering flowers after a funeral is over. Think of the beauty of the flowers as a final gift from a stranger who even in death can touch our lives. Taken apart and put in vases, they can fill the room with beauty and fragrance.

Holiday items can include hats and noisemakers for New Year's, valentines, Easter eggs and flowered Easter hats for the women, Passover items, Fourth of July flags, pictures of Thanksgiving, and Christmas ornaments to help residents recall past holiday events. I look to the activity department to help make sure seasonal and holiday items are kept current.

## MATTHEW'S STORY

Matthew began the day by being gently awakened by the care partner assigned to him. He was changed, dressed, and groomed while the care partner talked about Matthew's wife and children. After breakfast, Matthew was taken to the Namaste Care room, where soft and comforting music was playing. He was greeted by the Namaste Carer, taken from his wheelchair, and placed in a comfortable lounge chair close to the window. Matthew expressed how much he liked looking at the mountains when he was still able to communicate, so placing him near the window was a way to honor his wishes. A quilt was tucked around him, and small pillows were placed around him to ensure maximum comfort based on an evaluation done by the rehabilitation therapist for how best to position Matthew for comfort and safety. Next to Matthew was an over-the-bed table with pictures of his family: one of his children, one wedding picture, and one recent picture walking on the beach with his wife, Celia.

During the morning activities, Matthew was gently awakened by the sound of a bird (from a stuffed bird that makes genuine bird calls) and by conversation from the Namaste Carer about his interest in golf. His favorite bird was a pheasant because it made a call that sounded like his name. Celia particularly enjoyed making the little stuffed bird chirp "ma-coo"; she would laugh and hug her "ma-coo."

A special treat for Matthew was getting shaved in the Namaste Care room. His chair would be placed near the sink. The Namaste Carer would greet him with a kiss on the cheek, then remark that he looked scruffy; he smiled. She told him that he was going to have a wonderful shave so that he would look handsome for his visit with Celia in the afternoon. After a barber cape was placed around his shoulders, the Namaste Carer gently washed his face with a wet, warm face cloth and then placed a small, wet, warm towel on his face. The next step was to tell him about the shaving cream that was going to be smoothed on his face. She continued to talk to him as he was shaved. When finished, the Namaste Carer washed his face to wipe off any remaining shaving cream. This was one of the most pleasurable experiences for Matthew; he really showed a positive reaction. Celia told us that as a business-man he was always well dressed and groomed in the morning and that Matthew shaved every morning, even on the weekend. Although Matthew could not shave himself anymore, he was honored by keeping this ritual intact.

Matthew was not consuming enough calories during meals, so the Namaste Care team made sure he had high-calorie snacks and bever-ages throughout the day. Matthew was known to have a sweet tooth, so he was often given a lollipop to suck on. He was taken to his room to be changed and then went to the dining room for lunch.

## MORNING PAPERWORK

When the residents have left the room, the Namaste Carer makes sure food supplies are stored and the room is tidied for the after-noon session. I suggest that an attendance record be maintained. Although it is a nursing program, participation in Namaste Care is usually care planned under activities. Some communities also use a checklist to show what activities have been used (Appendix D). I also recommend a journal or place where notes can be kept about the residents' preferences. This helps communication between Namaste Carers.

## AFTERNOONS IN NAMASTE CARE

The Namaste Care room reopens after lunch for the afternoon activities, which differ somewhat from the morning program. Resi-dents attend both sessions unless they are having a medical problem and need to be taken to their room to rest or nursing determines that they must be repositioned in bed to maintain good skin integrity. Residents with advanced dementia will sleep most of the time, but at least in the Namaste Care room they are not alone and are receiving some individual attention. They may need to be changed and groomed after lunch before being taken to the Namaste Care room for afternoon programming.

The room is prepared for the afternoon the same way it was for the morning program, with the scent of lavender, dim lighting, and calming music. Everyone is welcomed back and made comfortable. Residents who did not attend the morning program will have their hands and faces washed and moisturized and their hair combed. Residents who attended the morning session will have different activities offered to them in the afternoon.

A large-screen television might be playing a movie classic or comedy show from the past, such as *I Love Lucy* for residents who seem to be more alert. Residents also seem to like videos of children and baby animals, or if it is a day when they need a more relaxing DVD, rainforest scenes are soothing. The splashes of color and movement of waterfalls or animals seem to attract the attention of some residents. Resources for activity supplies can be found in Appendix B.

## SOFT, FUN, FURRY, AND FAMILIAR

Each afternoon, the Namaste Carer or activity professional visits with each resident using a variety of items to explore ways to connect with him or her. Different fabrics, such as cashmere, silk, velvet, and rabbit fur, stimulate reactions. Used clothing, such as evening gowns, usually produces smiles from the women; perhaps they are recalling their younger days, when they went to dances dressed in their finest. Prom dresses and wedding gowns are inexpensive when purchased at second-hand stores, or you can ask for donations from families in the facility newsletter. Tuxedos and leather jackets for the men provide opportunities to recall special occasions. Hanging these supplies on a coat rack or draping them on a chair helps give the room a warm, homey feel. I often put a hat rack in the Namaste Care room and change the hats according to the season: sun hats and baseball caps in the summer and stocking caps, earmuffs, and scarves in the winter are reminders of the season and make the room look homier.

Some inexpensive and fun items that are simple but effective in producing chuckles include colorful pinwheels, fans, puppets, colorful small balls, and even chattering fake teeth. Singing Santa Claus figures and a plastic globe that snows when shaken always make residents smile. Sports items including golf equipment, basketballs, baseballs, uniform jerseys, and pictures of famous sports figures may be enjoyable, depending on the resident's level of awareness and interests. Keep trying different items until one creates a positive response.

*JOE*

> According to his family, Joe was an avid Red Sox fan. Staff decided to reach Joe through his love of the game. When a baseball glove and ball, a Red Sox hat, and pictures of sports figures he had admired were placed on a table near him, he became a happy man. He would smile and hold the baseball and glove, caressing the leather. Joe was basically unable to communicate, so imagine how surprised the Namaste Care team members were when he joined in a chorus of "Take Me Out to the Ball Game."

Residents with advanced dementia can still have smiles and laughter in their lives, but producing these bits of brightness takes some thought on the part of the Namaste Carer. They need to know what item will produce these happy moments. For instance, Betty's family informed us that she was a woman who "did lunch." She was unable to speak but positively beamed when we put her beautiful hat and white gloves on. Muriel loved having an evening gown draped around her, and Michael held tightly to his University of Michigan football sweater. Sometimes families are helpful, and other times we just keep trying different items until we find one that works.

RANGE OF MOTION

Residents involved in Namaste Care have lost the ability to exercise independently; they cannot follow directions and rarely move their hands and legs. In the afternoon, Namaste Carers engage residents in passive range-of-motion exercises to provide touch, help prevent contractures, and get the blood circulating. A physical therapist should show care partners how to make this activity pleasant and beneficial for the residents. Passive range-of-motion exercise includes slow movement of the hands, fingers, arms, feet, and legs.

During range-of-motion activities, care partners must continually assess the resident's facial reactions and verbal sounds for signs of discomfort. This is one of those times when several pairs of hands can work wonders. Educate family members to do range-of-motion exercises, and encourage them to visit during this activity time. To make exercising more fun, play upbeat music. With the room filled with some big-band sounds or a march, the residents can be placed in a circle while team members move from one resident to another providing range-of-motion stimulation and explaining what each procedure will involve. Even if a resident does not seem to understand what is being said, it is the Namaste Care way to explain every move to them.

Exercise can also be done with guided imagery. Tell a story and use a resident's arms and hands to describe the image. Say, "Let's look at how the sun is rising in the morning," and raise their arms as high as they will go without pain. Then talk about the breeze ruffling leaves in the trees and flutter the fingers. Residents in Honolulu do the hula to native music and the scent of gardenias.

Some residents may also be able to toss a ball back and forth, bat a balloon, or reach out for bubbles, the bigger the better. These are all very pleasant ways to exercise, and the activity department will have balls the Namaste Carer can try.

## HAND MASSAGE

I used to think giving a hand massage was simply washing the residents' hands and applying lotion to them. Then I met Lorna Reid, a nurse with ACCORD Hospice in Scotland who showed me the art of hand massage and gave me a copy of *Comforting Touch in Dementia and End of Life Care*, by Barbara Goldschmidt and Niamh van Meines. The book gives the background of touch therapy and many stories of residents with dementia who have benefited from touch.

The step-by-step instructions for what the authors describe as a "comforting touch session" can only be summarized here; the book is worth buying. The session begins with hand washing for both the giver and receiver. I'm using the term *massage*, but I do not mean to imply that this activity can be offered only by a licensed massage therapist. The authors suggest that at least 30 minutes should be allocated for each hand rub, and that would be difficult if not impossible for the Namaste Carer with 10 to 12 residents in the room. A more practical application is to teach this activity to volunteers, families, and other team members. When Lorna demonstrated the hand rub to me and other care partners, we could feel the effects after a 10-minute demonstration. The sequence recommended by Goldschmidt and van Meines is as follows and every gesture is repeated three times:

- Be present and in the moment, then apply soft, fluttering strokes that say "hello."
- Rub the shoulder and elbow with circular motions.
- Place the resident's hand with the palm facing down on your hand and make small circular strokes over the knuckles.
- Using your thumb, make gliding strokes over the top of the hand.
- Turn the hand over and rub the inside of the palm.
- Hold the hand and stroke down the fingers.
- Stroke the fingertips.
- Say goodbye by repeating the soft, fluttering strokes you began with.

## FOOT WASHING AND MASSAGE

What is now known as hospice care dates back to the days of the Knights of the Round Table. It seems that when they were too old to fight battles, they retired and were given the responsibility of caring for the oldest, sickest knights. The description of how care was provided to the dying is as current today as it was hundreds of years ago. Tales speak of providing clean linens, feeding warm soup, and washing the feet of the knights they cared for. There are also descriptions of Jesus washing the feet of the disciples. Foot washing is a humbling task and a loving gesture. In the Namaste Care room, foot washing is part of the day's ritual.

Foot massages are given using a careful and gentle touch, especially when rubbing over bony areas. The resident's feet are soaked one at a time in a basin with warm water and antibacterial soap, gently washed and dried, and massaged with lotion up to the knee. This procedure not only feels good but provides an opportunity for the Namaste Carer to assess the integrity of the residents' skin and the condition of their toenails. Nursing staff are immediately informed of any questionable areas on the leg or foot. Toenails must be trimmed by a podiatrist, so except for the cleaning and moisturizing they are left alone. The reaction of residents to this very basic and loving experience is an expression of complete bliss.

## OTHER SOUNDS OF MUSIC

Music is an important part of the Namaste Care program, not only the music that fills the air but also other items that make pleasantly stimulating sounds. The soft tinkling of a small wind chime, soft-sounding drums, triangles, and hand bells are a few of the ways to produce enjoyable musical sounds. These supplies have motion and make pleasant sounds. So many simple little objects are perfect for Namaste Care and well within the budget.

Rain sticks come in a variety of sizes and make beautiful soothing sounds; they can be found in most activity supply catalogs. Another stimulating instrument is the singing bowl. It is more difficult to find but very interesting to use. The bowls make a humming sound that resonates throughout the room. Music boxes are so much fun, and residents usually recognize their songs and tinkling sound. In the best of all possible worlds, the facility would employ the services of a music therapist. These are professionals who are very effective working in hospice and palliative care programs. Registered music therapists can be located through the yellow pages or on the Internet. The U.S. web site is www.musictherapy.org.

## NOURISHMENTS

Nourishments such as lollipops and juice are again offered in the afternoon. Make the afternoon special by also offering a treat such as soft ice cream or pudding. Some residents take pleasure in munching on a soft cookie that is easy to swallow and pleasurable to eat. Residents with advanced dementia usually retain a sweet tooth, so anything sweet is usually enjoyable and provides much-needed calories. Beverages are offered on a continuous basis, as they are in the morning. I discovered that in the United Kingdom tea is served every day at about 3 P.M. When the residents hear the tea trolley, they usually wake up; the sound must stir memories of days past. I am always amazed when residents who need someone to hold a cup for them to drink juice suddenly become very independent and hold their own teacup!

## MORE WAYS TO ENGAGE RESIDENTS

### Namaste à la Carte

Residents who are not physically able to leave their bed or choose not to be taken to the Namaste Care room can have the program come to them. With a bit of humor this is called Namaste à la carte. Nursing facilities are finding that the power of loving touch is important for almost all residents, and a cart is available for team members to use for in-room visits. Hospice staff can also use the items on the cart when they make visits to patients and their families. When a resident is actively dying, the cart is filled with items appropriate for families and staff to use when a person is in the last stage of life. (Refer to the No One Dies Alone program in Chapter 9.)

The cart should look like something residents would have in their homes. It must have drawers or shelves for storage and wheels so that it can easily be rolled into a resident's room. I have found great buys in furniture store clearance sections and discovered that wheels can be installed on almost anything. The look should be in keeping with honoring the spirit within, so we do not use institutional laundry or dietary carts. Colorful placemats on the top of the cart, fresh or silk flowers in a vase, and supplies stored in baskets are just some of the ways to make the cart useful yet attractive. Assemble a cart with the following materials:

- Lavender linen spray
- Lotions for hands and feet, scented and unscented
- A variety of seasonal scents
- Sensory items such as realistic birds, a music box, pictures
- CD player and a variety of music
- Hand wipes
- Plastic gloves
- Sensory items and fun items
- Religious items
- A variety of reading materials (e.g., religious or spiritual, familiar poems)

Residents will have combs and brushes in their rooms and personal items that can be used for reminiscence, such as pictures and greeting cards. Items can be borrowed from the Namaste Care room's supplies for afternoon visits. Residents may also be offered food and beverages, but care must be taken to follow dietary procedures for food handling.

Some nursing facilities place a cart on each floor to use when a resident is having problems sleeping or when someone is actively dying. Another creative idea is to put a lounge chair and the cart near the nurses' station. When a resident is wandering at night, invite him or her to sit in the "spa" chair, use the lavender linen spray on a blanket, and play soft music, and the wandering resident may be comfortable enough to fall asleep.

If a resident is in bed for long periods of time and bed rails are used, cover the bed rails with soft material to encourage tactile exploration (Calkins, 2005). Placing realistic stuffed animals in bed and long pillows on each side of the resident may help him or her feel secure and comforted. The important thing to remember is that Namaste Care is portable.

## RELIGION AND SPIRITUALITY

Meeting the religious needs of residents with advanced dementia is challenging because when they are taken to a service or mass, residents usually fall asleep. At this point in their lives, they need religious items, songs, hymns, and chants to help them reconnect with their religion. Once again, the Namaste Carer must know the religious history of the resident to make these activities personal and appropriate. This can be tricky because a person's family may say their loved one is not religious, and that may be true of the resident's adult life. However, the resident may have a history of being raised in a certain religion, and as the dementia progresses that is what he or she remembers. I created two bags to keep religious supplies in for Seasons Hospice. One had a cross (Protestant) and a crucifix (Catholic) on the front, the other a Jewish star, easy to do with iron-on or stenciled symbols. The following items were included in the bags:

- Cross and crucifix

- Rosary

- Bible, Catholic and Protestant

- Statue of the Blessed Mary

- Religious pictures

- Mezuzah

- Menorah

- Yarmulke

- CDs of hymns, songs, and chants

When a resident of another religion became part of Namaste Care, the family was asked to help provide items that their loved one could relate to. They were kept in a special storage container for that particular resident unless several residents shared that religion, then the facility would purchase the appropriate items.

Clergy were invited to come into the Namaste Care room to offer individual visits, and if the resident could safely swallow, communion was offered. Religious activities were offered on Sunday to Protestants and Catholics. For the Jewish residents, Friday Shabbat and Saturday activities became part of the weekend programs.

## INVOLVING THE FAMILY

Families often visit in the afternoon and must be politely cautioned that entering the room with a boisterous greeting and loud voice do not fit with the serenity of the Namaste Care afternoon program. A bit of sensitivity education helps team members and families understand that they must enter the Namaste Care room as a breeze softly flutters in a window, changing the feel of a room but not adding to or detracting from the atmosphere.

Family visits are sometimes difficult when their loved one is not able to speak and may not recognize the family members. Some family members, especially spouses, visit almost every day; their lives may be very empty with their husband or wife living apart from them. Sometimes they just do not know what to do during the visit. Something simple, such as giving a spouse hand cream to massage into their loved one's hand, can help connect them as a couple once again. In the United Kingdom a daughter was in tears when her mother began to massage her hand (Simard, 2012b). Another resident loved having his wife and daughter hold a lollipop for him to suck on, because he could no longer hold it himself. For some family members, especially spouses, visiting in Namaste Care gives them an opportunity for socialization with Namaste Carers and other residents' families. Namaste Care team members become a close extended family when they show support to very lonely spouses. Some adult children also have a sense of responsibility to care for their parents and feel guilty that they had to move them to a nursing facility. When they can still do something for them, such as brushing their mother's hair or giving dad his favorite ice cream, daughters and sons feel as if they can still provide something special for their parents. Families appreciate seeing that Namaste Carers take such good care of the person they love. From our research projects, and from what is communicated verbally and in letters of appreciation from families, we have found that families visit for longer periods of time and their visits are more enjoyable in the Namaste Care room.

With some assistance from Namaste Carers, most of the meaningful activities can be offered by families, such as brushing hair and giving hand massages. We also encourage families to bring things from home that may elicit a response from the resident. Families are Namaste Care guests, so offering them something to eat or drink when offering beverages to their loved one is an appropriate and courteous gesture.

Families should also be informed that they can take their loved one out of the room, perhaps to attend a music program or for a walk. My grandson, Justin, was 6 or 7 years old when he visited his 103-year-old great-grandmother. He was so proud that he was allowed to push her in the wheelchair. Justin still treasures that memory. Namaste Carers make sure that both the resident and family are in a safe situation when leaving the Namaste Care room. Many of the spouses are frail themselves and cannot manage wheelchairs without some assistance.

## MATTHEW'S STORY

After lunch, Matthew was toileted and either put to bed or taken back to the Namaste Care room. Matthew was again warmly greeted by the Namaste Carer. Many days he was not placed in a lounge chair because his wife was coming to visit, and she wanted to be able to wheel his chair outside or be alone with him. To prepare for her visit, Matthew was told she would be visiting, and a scarf with Celia's favorite perfume scent was placed around his neck. He loved Frank Sinatra and Dean Martin CDs, so he might have earphones with the songs he loved playing.

Celia arrived to hugs from care partners. They told her about Matthew's morning and all the positives they could communicate. As his condition deteriorated, it was important for her to hear that he was happy and well cared for. Like so many spouses, Celia had cared for Matthew for many years, and it was difficult to turn his care over to others and to live without him. The Namaste Carers were very affectionate, and Celia got a healthy dose of hugs whenever she visited.

During the afternoon, Matthew had range-of-motion exercises. He seemed to enjoy a variety of musical sounds such as a rain stick, bells, or wind chimes. He especially liked chocolate pudding; his eyes glowed when the pudding arrived, and either Celia or the Namaste Carer fed him.

Sometimes Namaste Carers just held his hand and looked into his eyes. Matthew was loved, and with his peaceful demeanor, we believe he felt it. Namaste Care programming ended before the evening meal. Again Matthew was toileted and taken to the dining room, then readied for bed. Music he especially liked was played on a bedside tape deck. He was well cared for throughout the day, with good nursing care and meaningful activities that enhanced his life.

## END OF DAY

The Namaste Care Room closes before the evening meal with lively music and the lights turned up. Each resident is bid farewell with a touch. "Thank you for joining me this afternoon" and a hug are a perfect way to end the day for the resident and the staff. After the room is empty, the Namaste Carer makes sure all soiled laundry is taken to the laundry room and the room is readied for the next morning by turning off appliances, wiping counters, checking food supplies, tossing out-of-date items, and so forth. Paperwork is completed, the Namaste Care room is gently closed, and the day is done.

I'm reminded of a Girl Scout song we would end the day with, sung to the tune of "Taps":

> Day is done, gone the sun
> From the lakes, from the hills, from the sky.
> All is well, safely rest. God is nigh.

# CHAPTER 6

# *Implementing Namaste Care*

Begin with the end in mind.

STEPHEN COVEY

In his book *The Seven Habits of Highly Effective People*, Stephen Covey's second habit is "begin with the end in mind." This is a perfect way to begin thinking about your Namaste Care™ program. Is the "end" a vision that will establish your facility as specialist in dementia care? Most nursing facilities and assisted living communities offer the same services; what makes yours unique? Do you even have a niche? If Namaste Care is the catalyst for your vision to be the facility of choice for families and other referral sources looking for dementia care, the implementation plan should be more comprehensive because the entire organization needs to be involved in the process and feel a part of the vision for your niche. Or do you need a "quick fix" after experiencing survey problems that a Namaste Care program may help to resolve? If that is true, the implementation process may need to be accelerated. When you have decided what the "end" will be, a plan for the implementation process can be developed.

I prefer to describe this as a vision plan. I like this term because it brings a fresh approach to doing something out of the ordinary. The first step in developing the vision plan is to decide on the scope of the program: Will it be a day program or a neighborhood? When this decision has been made, the timeline for implementation can be developed. It should be flexible so that even in the planning stage and implementation process, Namaste Care is a joy, not a just another project.

The implementation of Namaste Care begins with selling the program to the decision maker, usually the administrator, in your nursing facility. This is assuming that you, the reader, are not the decision maker. Request a meeting with the administrator, during which you will be undisturbed and preferably away from a telephone. Offer this book or information from it, before the meeting or as part of your presentation, and personalize the program to your facility. Use examples of real residents to show how Namaste Care will benefit the facility's residents. These touches help to make the program real, not a theoretical concept.

One administrator was swayed to advocate for Namaste Care by "the rabbi's" story. The rabbi, once a well-known and respected member of the local religious community, was in the advanced stage of Alzheimer's disease. This resident tugged on the heartstrings of the administrator and staff as they witnessed the toll Alzheimer's disease was taking on him. He looked so frail and lonely. Here is his story:

## THE RABBI

His eyes were haunting. Most days the rabbi was in a lounge chair or in bed with a feeding tube that provided continuous nutrition. Often, a soap opera or *The Jerry Springer Show* was on the television set— the staff's choice, definitely not his. The rabbi was clearly well cared for, with clean clothes and his yarmulke firmly in place. He was in the advanced stage of Alzheimer's disease, was nonambulatory, and needed total care; except for strong eye contact, he was nonverbal. The rabbi rarely left his room because of his feeding tube. He did not participate in any activities other than occasional religious services, when he was wheeled into the room with his feeding tube equipment. Someone had to sit with him so that no other resident would touch the feeding tube. The activity department visited him several times each week and read passages from religious books, nurses took care of his physical needs, and occasionally he had a visitor. That left hours alone. What kind of quality of life was this for a man who had dedicated his life to others?

His physician determined that he could go for periods of time without the feeding tube. Nursing agreed that if he had a place to go, he could be taken off the feeding tube for these periods. In Namaste Care, the rabbi would not be alone. He would be with others and would benefit from the activities that were still meaningful to him. Namaste Carers would talk to him, recalling his life's work that was so important to him and the community he served. He could listen to favorite religious music and chants that had been a major source of pleasure in his life. Music would be played for him on headphones or played for everyone in the Namaste Care room. The rabbi would be part of the Namaste Care community; he would be in the presence of others, as he had been throughout most of his life.

When the rabbi was taken to his room for tube feeding, Namaste Care continued. Favorite music, as identified by his family, would be played or a video of religious services would be shown on his television. The cable would be disconnected, and there would be no more soap operas or Jerry Springer.

Creating a story of how life would change for the rabbi helped convince the administrator that Namaste Care should be implemented and become part of a new vision, to be the very best provider of dementia services in the marketplace.

Administrators want the best possible quality of life for their residents, but they also have fiscal responsibility for the facility. The next logical question from the administrator is usually, "How much will this cost?" Therefore, it is important to develop a budget that includes expenses and a projected increase in revenue.

## DEVELOPING A BUDGET

The kiss of death for any proposed new program is to suggest that care partners need to be added to the budget. Adding team members to provide Namaste Care, at least in the beginning of the program, is not necessary. In most facilities, one care partner from the dementia care neighborhood is designated as the Namaste Carer and is assigned to the Namaste Care room for the morning shift and one for the afternoon shift, or they have responsibility for the day. When the Namaste Carer is in the room, other care partners monitor the residents assigned to them who are not in the room. (Additional ideas regarding Namaste Care team members and the Namaste Care day can be found in Chapters 3 and 5, respectively.)

If the decision is made to add a dedicated Namaste Carer, their hours are usually 9 to 4:30. The Namaste Care room is open from 9:30 A.M. until 11:30 A.M., or whenever lunch is served. It reopens at 2:00 P.M., or when residents have been fed and changed. The room usually closes at 4:00 P.M. The half hour before opening and after closing gives Namaste Carers time to gather supplies and ready the room for their residents. It also allows time at the end of the day for charting and preparing the room for the next day. The Namaste Care program takes place 7 days per week. The salary that a Namaste Carer receives should be higher than that of a care partner, activity assistant, or restorative aide. This provides an incentive for team members to consider taking this position and gives them another career option. Additional information on the Namaste Carer can be found in Chapter 3.

## CENSUS PROJECTIONS

Follow these steps to project how much additional revenue you can expect to receive from additional facility residents:

- Assess the existing dementia care program and decide whether residents who no longer need the security of a dementia care neighborhood can be relocated to another area of the facility where a new Namaste Care neighborhood could be located. This would free up beds in the secured neighborhood that could be filled with new admissions to the dementia program.

- Meet with local hospice programs to determine whether Namaste Care would increase referrals from them.

- Meet with referral sources; explain the purpose of Namaste Care and elicit feedback from them about the need for this type of program.

- Visit your competition to determine whether adding Namaste Care would provide a program not offered by other nursing facilities or assisted living communities in your area.

New programs often have a trickle-down effect. Even though a family might not need Namaste Care for their loved one when they move in, they may recognize the value of a facility offering this unique type of program.

## PHYSICAL PLANT COSTS

The Namaste Care program may take place in a space used solely for the program or in a room that is shared and used for other purposes when Namaste Care program is not scheduled. When it is a dedicated room, strive to give the room a warm, comforting look. It is amazing what a coat of paint and a wallpaper border can do to improve the look of a room. Some facilities start small, first locating their Namaste Care program in a vacant resident room or the conference room. I will never forget Jay Brooks, executive director at Brethren Village in Ashland, Ohio. Jay asked me to consult with his facility to implement Namaste Care. His facility had no extra space that I could deem suitable, and, believe me, I can usually find space. We met with his team, trying to come up with a solution, and one brave member of his team suggested that the only large space that was not well used was the conference room we were meeting in. An administrator giving up a conference room would never happen, or so I thought. Jay paused for a minute, then said, "You are right." Within a month, the large conference table was in storage, the team held meetings in the dining room, and Namaste Care was changing the lives of 10 residents.

When the administrator sees how many residents need the program, a larger space to accommodate more residents is usually found. Startup expenses will differ depending on what is needed but may include the following:

- Paint and wallpaper border
- Emergency call system for team members (e.g., a wall call bell, telephone, or handheld device)
- Removal (or disabling) of any overhead paging systems
- Window coverings that filter direct sunlight and look attractive
- Heating and cooling system that can maintain the room at a comfortable temperature for residents who are frail and usually cold

- Flooring that can be cleaned easily and does not have a high gloss
- Sink for hand washing
- Refrigerator
- Soap and towel dispensers
- Music system
- Television set with DVD
- Nursing supplies (see Appendix A)
- Quilts or blankets
- Secured storage for supplies
- Reclining lounge chairs. This is the biggest expense, although in skilled facilities many residents will already have a wheelchair that reclines. In assisted living communities where they do not want a "nursing home look," families may provide the chairs. Hospice patients can get a lounge chair as part of the Medicare hospice benefit, but finding one that is acceptable for assisted living is a challenge.
- Small tables (over-the-bed tables will work) for residents' personal items
- Chairs for visitors
- Storage for individual resident quilts and personal care items
- Namaste cart

Additional information on decorating the Namaste Care room can be found in Chapter 4. Lists of activity supplies, such as rain sticks and other sensory items, can be found in Appendix B. Sources for these supplies can be found in Appendix C.

## MANAGEMENT TEAM

When the budget has been approved by the administrator and a green light has been given to go forward, the management team must be convinced to support the program. It is difficult or impossible to start Namaste Care without their support. The entire management team needs to be knowledgeable about the Namaste Care concept, and their input must be requested and acknowledged.

The director of nursing (DON) is at the top of the list of people who must agree to the program in order for it to be successful. Namaste Care is primarily a nursing responsibility; in fact, DONs have called it an enhanced nursing program. The DON is responsible for Namaste Care; however, the day-to-day supervision of the program is often delegated to the assistant director of nursing (ADON). It is important that whoever supervises Namaste Care sees the program at least once a day to ensure that all regulations and infection control requirements are addressed and to monitor behavioral changes of residents who are on any type of antipsychotic medication. On weekends, this responsibility is assigned to the nursing supervisor. One of the goals of Namaste Care is to eliminate or at least decrease the need for this type of medication, so the presence of nursing is extremely important. They are the ones who call the physician regarding decreasing or eliminating medications. Other members of the management team need to be supportive because they all have a role in the success of the Namaste Care program or neighborhood. Ideas for how their particular expertise is needed include the following:

- The life enrichment director (activities) provides some help by assigning team members to assist with Namaste Care and suggests supplies and new program ideas.

- The director of maintenance is responsible for making renovations to the Namaste Care room and ensuring that all equipment is in compliance with fire and safety codes.

- The director of housekeeping is responsible for keeping the Namaste Care room supplied with linen and maintaining the room in a clean and safe condition.

- The director of marketing is responsible for marketing the program to referral sources and generating positive public relations.

- The director of admissions is responsible for explaining Namaste Care to new families.

- The director of social work is responsible for helping family members understand how Namaste Care can provide quality-of-life programming for their loved one.

- The director of food services is responsible for providing food and beverages on a daily basis and ensuring that sanitary regulations are followed.

- The director of staff development is responsible for organizing team members, educating family members, and incorporating Namaste Care into the orientation of all new employees.

Many of these positions are not found in assisted living communities. Refer to Chapter 7 for information on how these responsibilities are assigned in assisted living.

As part of the buy-in process, the administrator should schedule a meeting with all department managers to explain the Namaste Care program. Before this meeting it is helpful to have department managers read the Namaste Care book so that they have some idea about the program and have thought about the impact it may have on their department. After the initial meeting to disseminate information and answer questions, the administrator and department managers develop a plan for implementation. Some administrators prefer to form a smaller group of managers to develop the implementation plan and then present it to all managers for their input.

## IMPLEMENTATION PLAN

With the backing of the management team, the implementation process begins. A good plan is one that is flexible enough to change as needed. A sample implementation schedule follows:

1. Schedule an information and education meeting with all team members to explain Namaste Care. This meeting may include educational information on Alzheimer's disease. Educating all team members employed in the facility about Alzheimer's disease is one of the first steps in making sure that the facility is dementia friendly. Many states now require Alzheimer's disease training for staff at least once a year, so this step will help meet this requirement.

2. Insert a letter into team members' pay envelopes explaining Namaste Care for those who could not attend the meetings and reinforce what was explained at the meeting. Translate this letter into other languages as necessary.

3. Meet with local hospice programs and other referral agencies to explain the program.

4. Schedule a family meeting to explain Namaste Care and answer any questions.

5. Follow up this meeting with a letter to families or an article in the facility's newsletter.

6. Schedule a meeting with alert, oriented residents to discuss Namaste Care and answer their questions.

7. Decide on the location of the Namaste Care room and any other special rooms associated with the program, such as the Reagan Room (a private room for actively dying residents; see Chapter 4).

8. Interview team members who may want to work in the program.

9. Select and hire Namaste Carers or team members.

10. Provide special education for the Namaste Carers who will lead the daily program.

11. Purchase supplies and equipment.

12. Make the physical plant changes in the Namaste Care room.

13. Identify potential residents for the program and approach their families.

14. Determine a start date for services.

15. Issue a press release on Namaste Care.

16. Schedule to make extra team members available on the opening day.

17. Plan an opening celebration; include all team members, families, residents, referral sources, and the media.

After Namaste Care has been introduced, the energy surrounding it will carry the implementation through the challenges that always surface when something new is started in a nursing facility.

## INTERNAL MARKETING

Internal marketing is highly important. It is a mistake to implement a new program or make major changes without letting all team members know what you are doing. Rumors begin flying, and misinformation is difficult to wipe away. There are many ways to let team members know as soon as the decision has been made to go forward with Namaste Care.

### Introducing Namaste Care to Team Members

Informing all team members in the facility, taking into account days off, sick days, and vacations, is a challenge. A mandatory meeting for all team members is recommended but may not be feasible because of the high cost of bringing in team members when they are not scheduled to work. Also, many employees have two jobs or have child care responsibilities that make attending a special meeting outside their shifts difficult or impossible. An alternative is to schedule several short 30-minute meetings during a 2- or 3-day period. Assign one or two people to lead the meetings, thereby providing a consistent message. If another facility in your company has a Namaste Care program, you might want to have staff visit so they can see the actual program and give their impression to other team members.

Even after this initial educational meeting, the person responsible for the orientation of new employees should integrate Namaste Care information into all orientation in-services. Here are some creative ideas on how to educate team members:

- Hold a special in-service and award a certificate to all those attending. Ring a chime or singing bowl to begin the meeting. The magical sound creates a dramatic beginning to the presentation.

- Provide education during a working lunch for each department; serve food during the presentation and use the opportunity to personally thank all team members for how they care for and about the residents, their families, and each other.

- Pamper team members with Namaste Care supplies and activities. Give hand massages, (see Chapter 5), play soothing music, and distribute lollipops to simulate some of the meaningful activities offered to residents during the Namaste Care day.

## OUTLINE OF TEAM MEMBERS' IN-SERVICE

The following outline describes how information on Namaste Care, as well as Alzheimer's disease, can be presented to the team members.

### Introduction

A speaker, usually the administrator or director of nursing, introduces himself or herself and informs the team members of the purpose of the meeting. Team members are provided with handouts that include a brief description of Namaste Care and an outline of the daily programs.

### Overview of Alzheimer's Disease

Review basic information about Alzheimer's disease, including risk factors, warning signs, diagnosis, treatments, stages, and behavior symptoms related to the stages. Discuss the benefits and burdens of cardiopulmonary resuscitation, hospitalization, treatment of infections, tube feeding, catheters, and medications. The Alzheimer's Association's web site is a wonderful resource to use for this in-service (www.alz.org/index.asp).

### Comfort Care

Spend time emphasizing the importance of comfort care for these residents. Explain to team members the Namaste Care philosophy on clothing, lounge chairs, bathing, and grooming. Review how to assess a resident with advanced dementia for pain and discomfort.

### Namaste Care

This book can be used as an outline for a Namaste Care in-service. Explaining the meaning and philosophy of Namaste Care and describing a typical day, with a team member playing a resident, is very effective way to educate team members. You can create a Namaste Care atmosphere so that when team members come into the in-service, they can feel the difference. Dim the lights, spray the room with lavender, and play music. It is also a good idea to offer an example of a resident in your facility and how he or she might benefit from Namaste Care, something like the previous story of the rabbi. I sometimes ask team members whether they can think of any resident who might be appropriate for Namaste Care, and we all brainstorm how their lives would change with Namaste Care.

Sometimes the changes are dramatic. For instance, in one care home I visited in the London area, a woman had been bedbound for 5 years with severe contractures. When they started a Namaste Care program, team members realized that with a proper chair she could be taken to the Namaste Care room, where she would no longer be isolated. Her son visited the day her chair arrived, and when he saw his mother in a room with other residents, having a gentle massage, he broke down and cried with happiness. Another care home, this one in Australia, had the use of a large room for their program. When they started their Namaste Care program, team members decided that a woman who had been bedbound for skin breakdown and was treated with a special air mattress could be wheeled into the room to be part of the program. This made a significant difference in her quality of life. "There are those that look at things the way they are, and ask why? I dream of things that never were, and ask why not?" This quote from Robert Kennedy reminds me to trust team members to help establish the vision plan for their facility.

At this point in the vision plan, you will know whether the Namaste Carer will be a new position or one that is shared. This information will be very important to explain to team members, especially if it will be added to their job description. You will also want to tell team members that if anyone is particularly interested or wants more information about the Namaste Care position, they should speak with their supervisor or whoever you have designated as the contact person. Team members will also be interested in knowing when the program is scheduled to open.

The in-service usually lasts 45 minutes; allow another 15 minutes for questions and comments. Encourage participation by asking whether the team members can see how Namaste Care would benefit particular residents. At the end of the in-service, give each team member a lollipop, a Namaste Care hallmark.

## Huddles

During the implementation of Namaste Care, all involved team members should be provided updates on a regular basis. These updates offer an opportunity for Namaste Carers and other team members to hear about the progress of the program and the next steps in the implementation process and for administrators not only to quash any rumors but solicit questions and suggestions from everyone. This can also provide a forum to thank all team members for their help in making Namaste Care a reality. I call these sessions huddles: brief meetings scheduled at a time when most of the team members are present but no privacy issues are discussed. Here are some good opportunities to call a huddle:

- Waiting for lunch to be delivered. No one is on break or at lunch; nurses and care partners are usually gathered in the dining room, where residents are assembled, waiting for the meal to be delivered, and housekeeping and activity team members can join the group in the dining room.

- During changes of shift

- During a large-scale resident entertainment program when most of the residents are occupied

- Any time that the nursing team members suggest; the team members have a better feel for what needs to be accomplished and when colleagues are available.

After Namaste Care has started, huddles can be held in the Namaste Care room with all the residents present as long as no private matters are discussed. A care partner from another neighborhood or someone from the management team can keep an eye on the residents during the huddle. This show of support from administration and the DON goes a long way in helping the care partners feel that Namaste Care is important.

Remember to keep meetings brief and avoid adding extra pressure or tasks for care partners. Include night team members in some huddles. Although these team members do not work during the hours when the programming occurs, it is important for them to feel included and knowledgeable about Namaste Care because the facility may have a Namaste Care cart that the evening and night shift could use if a resident is having problems sleeping or is actively dying. Keep huddles brief and positive. For any information that is not covered in a huddle, consider posting notices near the time clock; this ensures that all team members will see the postings.

Huddles offer an opportunity for team members to discuss what is going well and what challenges are occurring. During these meetings, new ideas will be generated that will make Namaste Care grow and make your facility's program unique. Namaste Care is like a butterfly, and a facility's team members give it wings.

## EVALUATION AND ONGOING COMMUNICATION

All facility team members should be encouraged to spend some time in the Namaste Care room when the program is in place so that they see for themselves the changes in residents. Often, care partners will learn from Namaste Carers about a particular activity a resident enjoys, such as hand massages, and will try doing this special activity on their own when they have a break in the day or if the resident becomes agitated. Namaste Care techniques are helpful for all team members to use for calming residents. After Namaste Care has officially begun, evaluation and ongoing communication must occur on a regular basis. At least once a month, Namaste Carers and other team members who work with the residents should have an opportunity to discuss the program. The team can be asked to recommend additional residents who would benefit from Namaste Care, keeping the program growing. Namaste Carers should also review the status of current residents and share what they know about activities each resident enjoys.

Mechanisms should be in place so that any administrator or department manager can evaluate the program to ensure its ongoing integrity. A Namaste Care checklist, for example, aids in this evaluation process (see Appendix D), ensuring that routine maintenance procedures are followed and supplies kept on hand. Oversight by the administrator or department manager should occur on at least a monthly basis. With the checklist in hand, they can make an evaluation of the program in a short period of time.

## INTRODUCING NAMASTE CARE TO FAMILIES

A special meeting should be scheduled to inform current family members about the plans to implement Namaste Care. They will begin to hear about it through the team members, so it is important to inform them as soon as possible after a decision has been made to implement the program. Family members, especially those who have a loved one with dementia, need to understand how Namaste Care is unique. If Namaste Care is going to be a dedicated neighborhood in the facility, make it clear that when residents with dementia reach the advanced stage of their disease, the facility team members may recommend a transfer to the neighborhood, but families make the final decision. Introducing Namaste Care to families provides the facility with an opportunity to educate family members on the medical issues that accompany the advanced stage of dementia, such as their loved one not eating or drinking as they were at an earlier stage of the disease and the medical burdens of tube feeding and hospitalization. Inviting a health care expert, hospice provider, or the facility medical director to give the presentation or to conduct part of the meeting is also a good way to attract families to attend.

Families are often a good resource for attracting new residents. A happy family member is the facility's best spokesperson. One support group leader, the spouse of a man in the advanced stage of Alzheimer's disease, went to her meeting excited about this new program offered at her husband's nursing facility. Rather than her usual tears, she enthusiastically spoke about Namaste Care and described the hand massage her husband was receiving when she visited. She said that she enjoyed this visit because the Namaste Carer gave her hand lotion to apply, and her usually unresponsive husband said, "I love you." This testimonial enticed another family member who attended the meeting to transfer her husband to this facility.

## INTRODUCING NAMASTE CARE TO RESIDENTS

The alert, oriented residents in a nursing facility are well attuned to their surroundings and need to know the details of Namaste Care. The president of the Resident Council should be informed about Namaste Care and a special meeting scheduled for residents. At the meeting, residents are told about Namaste Care, given written information on the program, and asked for their feedback.

The meeting can be enjoyable and educational by demonstrating hand massages and offering lollipops or ice cream to everyone. Residents should be encouraged to visit the Namaste Care room when it opens. This is also a time to recruit resident volunteers who may be willing to sit with residents in the Namaste Care room.

This resident meeting provides an opportunity to open related discussions about hospice care and advanced directives. These are topics that residents find less distressing to discuss than their family members do. A woman named Mary, who was in a great deal of pain and approaching the end of her life according to the nurses, expressed a common sentiment when I asked her whether she was afraid of dying. "Oh, no," she replied, "It's the living I fear!" Many residents report that they do not want to die in pain or alone, and most are just amazed at having lived so long. The residents who attend the meeting about the Namaste Care program seem comforted to know that this type of program is available to them if they need it.

## EXTERNAL MARKETING

### Public Relations

Public relations and the marketing of Namaste Care to the local community should begin as soon as the decision has been made to implement the program. A press release is a good way to inform the media of this new program; include information about the program and a contact number. Press releases must be followed up, especially if the object is to get coverage for an event such as the opening of the program or Namaste Care neighborhood. Media sources need reminders for several days leading up to the event. When the program is in place, media outlets can be invited to view the program and interview Namaste Care team members.

Invite the press to cover Namaste Care. This can be very positive, as long as you are well prepared. When the press is invited to the building, take measures to ensure that everything is sparkling. Remember that the overall impressions of the building, residents, team members, and care will influence the story reporters write and the pictures they take. Some Namaste Care neighborhoods have special T-shirts made for team members to wear for events such as this. Before a visit from the media you may want to send written material or speak to them, explaining what they will encounter. Residents with advanced dementia can be shocking to those who are unprepared.

Remember to inform the team members in advance that media personnel will be in the building. You may want to schedule an additional care partner to help get residents up and groomed, looking their best that day. Each resident in Namaste Care should always be well groomed; on a day when the media personnel are in the building, take extra care to have residents look their best. Housekeeping should also be advised, and, if necessary, schedule an extra person on that day in order to get the building in shape for the visitors. Take a walk outside the facility before the press arrives to make sure trash is picked up and landscaping is in good condition. I'll never forget one building I once toured. The dining room was nicely set with flowers on all the tables, but the flowers were all dead. Many years later, I still remember the image.

The Namaste Care room should be set up with Namaste Carers giving hand massages and providing sensory activities. When reporters see the activity in the room, witness the happy expressions of residents with lollipops in their mouths, hear the beautiful music, and smell the scent of lavender, they will have a true image of Namaste Care.

Remember to obtain photograph release forms from families before allowing the press to take pictures of residents or team members. Usually a verbal consent is sufficient for team members. Family members of Namaste Care residents may have strong feelings about having pictures taken of their loved one at this time of life. Inform photographers before they come to the facility about whom they can and cannot photograph or film. Some facilities will designate residents who cannot have their pictures taken by placing a sticker on their chair or on their clothing.

Giving interviews to the press is a great opportunity to tell the Namaste Care story. But remember that what is printed may be the impressions of the interviewer, not what the interviewee actually said. The person interviewed can ask to see a copy of the article before it is published, but this request is rarely granted. To avoid any surprises, prepare for an interview by developing a list of talking points. These are key responses to questions and what you want to communicate in the interview. Learn how to effectively develop talking points by watching a Sunday news program featuring a politician. They give five or six answers no matter what the question is.

Talking points for Namaste Care might include the following:

- The name of your facility

- The meaning of Namaste Care, "to honor the spirit within," as it relates to residents with advanced dementia

- The groundbreaking nature of the program

- The focus on providing improved quality-of-life programming for residents with advanced dementia

- The beauty of the Namaste Care room dedicated to the new program

- The special private room available for residents and families to be together at the end of a life

- The satisfaction of family members with Namaste Care and with the exceptional care their loved one is receiving

- The dedicated Namaste Carer (if you have hired additional staff)

The marketing team members can help draft these talking points, or they can be developed with input from the management team. A practice interview may help team members feel more comfortable. Following are some examples from my interviewing experiences. These show how to respond to an interviewer's harsh questions in order to establish your talking points and make the interview a positive experience.

*Interviewer:*  I understand that there is a great deal of abuse in nursing homes.

*Team member:*  We all deplore hearing about the few abuse stories that are in the news. Thank you for providing me with an opportunity to talk about Namaste Care, a new program at [nursing facility]. It is the first program in the city for residents with advanced dementia. We are proud of our reputation of providing excellent dementia care. Our newest program, Namaste Care, is another example of how we are constantly adding services to help our residents experience a high quality of life while they are with us.

*Interviewer:*  I understand this program is for people with advanced dementia who don't respond and can't remember anything. How do you know it makes a difference at this stage of their lives?

*Team member:*  Namaste Care means "to honor the spirit within," and we believe that every person has the right to excellent care in the presence of others throughout their lives. Not only does Namaste Care at [nursing facility] give residents this quality-of-life experience, but families tell us they feel a burden has been lifted when they walk into our beautiful Namaste Care room and see their loved one in a comfortable lounge chair, listening to beautiful music, receiving a hand massage, and sucking on a lollipop.

*Interviewer:*  So much has been in the news about finding a cure for Alzheimer's disease. Won't you lose a lot of money if a cure is found?

*Team member:* If a cure is found, we will be the first to celebrate. However, until that day arrives we will continue to provide excellent care for people with all stages of Alzheimer's disease. Namaste Care is a unique program in [city] to offer this type of care to residents with advanced dementia.

Most of the time, reporters are polite and the questions are fair. Even when questions seem leading, they can be turned around so that the facility comes across as caring and professional. I once did a call-in radio show. The very first caller told me that he had advised his family that he would kill himself if he was ever diagnosed with Alzheimer's disease. My reply was that receiving a diagnosis of any terminal disease is devastating (validating his feelings) and that now medications and lifestyle approaches may help to slow the disease process. New medications are being approved on a regular basis (offering hope), and the cure is closer. Then, to show him the fun that is experienced by residents with dementia, I told him about a recent visit to a dementia program where the residents were having a great time performing a selection of music for me on kazoos. I ended the call with an invitation to visit the facility and see for himself how people can live with the disease (extending hospitality) and thanked him for calling. Whew!

Most interviews are not this challenging, and most interviewers are very professional. It is a good idea to ask the interviewer how much time has been allocated for the interview. Knowing the time limitations will help you prioritize what to say. Also, ask whether the interviewer has any personal experience with someone who has Alzheimer's disease. Often, he or she has personal experience that can be related to the audience; this gives the interview a personal touch.

Television coverage is usually limited to a brief interview, so making sure you get all your talking points across is not easy. The interview is usually shown the same day it is filmed or the next day. Ask when it will be shown so that the show can be taped for marketing purposes. Tapes of any good news coverage, as well as newsprint articles, are a bonus to show during marketing events. After the coverage, be sure to send a thank-you note to the radio or television station or newspaper.

## REFERRAL SOURCES

Health care professionals who refer residents want the best care for their clients. When the decision is made to offer Namaste Care, marketing material should be developed for referral sources. Referral sources usually like the idea that the facility is providing something out of the ordinary and that the administration is willing to put money, time, and effort into enhancing the care given to residents. Marketing team members appreciate having something new to talk about during their calls to referral agencies. Agencies that may appreciate information on Namaste Care include the following:

- All referral sources currently in the facility marketing database
- The local chapter of the Alzheimer's Association or other groups devoted to Alzheimer's disease
- Alzheimer's support group leaders
- Area Agency on Aging
- Hospice programs
- Physicians
- Health maintenance organizations
- Senior referral agencies such as geriatric case managers
- Hospital discharge planners

An effective way to publicize Namaste Care is to offer a continuing education unit program. This is an effective way to get health care professionals to the facility. Programs such as Namaste Care that provide the latest research on end-of-life care provide interesting clinical information. It is very effective to schedule the program when Namaste Care is in place and to invite attendees to observe the program in small groups after the presentation. Usually the marketing team members like to provide small items to those attending the program. If possible, these gifts should be related to the presentation. For example, a Namaste Care gift bag could contain hand lotion, lavender sachets, chocolate, and lollipops. A door prize could be a service at a day spa or CDs of the soothing music played in the Namaste Care room. Food served may include smoothies or ice cream and of course lollipops! Implementing Namaste Care is a process that requires support from all team members. Helping the program reach as many residents as possible is an opportunity to educate the health care community and families who have loved ones with Alzheimer's disease that quality of life is possible for nursing home residents with advanced dementia and that your facility is leading the way in providing this special end-of-life care.

## MATTHEW'S STORY

Matthew's wife, Celia, was invited to a family meeting that was scheduled to provide an opportunity to describe Namaste Care to family members. This meeting was facilitated by the dementia program director, the charge nurse on the dementia neighborhood, and the charge nurse from the new Namaste Care neighborhood. They were able to answer questions from family members who were concerned that they would have to move their loved ones away from the neighborhood where they were familiar with the team members and happy with the care. It was reinforced that no one would be forced to move their loved one. Celia began to feel more comfortable that the excellent care Matthew was receiving would continue in the new wing. She was also very pleased to hear that Mary Longtin, the restorative aide who had begun what was now Namaste Care, would be leading the program on the new neighborhood. Rather than the few hours a week that Mary was offering her special activities to residents with advanced dementia, she was now going to be able to offer them at least 4 hours a day 7 days a week. Celia knew that Matthew's condition was deteriorating and that she would have to be prepared for a move to the new neighborhood in the near future. This meeting gave her a positive feeling about the care her husband would receive on the new wing, and she felt more comfortable after hearing the charge nurse talk about Namaste Care.

# CHAPTER 7

# Assisted Living

One person can make a
difference and every person should try.

JOHN FITZGERALD KENNEDY

When the first edition of this book was published in 2007, I did not believe that the majority of assisted living communities would be able to offer Namaste Care™ to their residents, and, as a matter of fact, assisted living was mentioned just a few times in the first edition. At that time, most residents were transferred to skilled nursing facilities when they reached the advanced stage of a dementing illness. That has changed, and residents in many states are allowed to stay in assisted living communities until death. Hence the need for a chapter devoted to the differences in implementing Namaste Care in assisted living as opposed to skilled nursing facilities.

In some states residents can stay in assisted living communities throughout the disease process because changes have been made in state regulations that allow them to care for residents with a higher level of acuity. More families are also electing the Medicare hospice benefit and, with the additional services and support they offer, assisted living communities can keep residents until death. In other situations, families choose to provide private duty nursing assistants to augment the community's carers. They would rather spend money on the extra staff than move their loved one to a nursing home. In many states, therefore, aging in place has become a reality for residents in assisted living.

Determining whether a resident with advanced dementia can stay in an assisted living community is complicated by regulations that differ from state to state; even the definition of assisted living is not universal, as some states license "rest homes" or "personal care homes." Assisted living is a state program, not a federal one, so there is not one set of regulations that apply to all communities. Individual states regulate what services can be provided under the various licenses. States can even designate who surveys the communities and how often the surveys take place.

There are also assisted living communities in both the United Kingdom and Australia, two countries where I have implemented Namaste Care. In the United Kingdom assisted living is licensed as residential care, and in Australia it is known as low care. American assisted living companies are opening communities in both countries, so the American model of care is being duplicated and the term *assisted living* is becoming more well known.

Since 2003, I have implemented Namaste Care in a few assisted living communities; however, I certainly did not possess the range of experiences in assisted living communities that I have in skilled nursing facilities. Then, I had the incredible good fortune in January 2012 to meet Pauline Coram, director of executive learning, and the dedicated people of Arden Courts, an assisted living company that specializes in dementia care ("Memory Care is all we do").

Arden Courts is part of HCR ManorCare, a large corporation providing a broad array of health care services. Often people from large corporations speak to me after Namaste Care presentations and tell me they see the need for Namaste Care but think they could never get it approved by all the corporate levels necessary in their communities. I understand. Having worked in many large corporations, I know that the time and energy needed to make a change occur in the organization is sometimes overwhelming, especially for managers and team members who are already overworked. The Arden Courts example in this chapter will show how to adapt the nursing home model of Namaste Care to an assisted living community and show how one person, even in a large corporation, can bring about change.

Debra Mittelbach, the executive director of Arden Courts in Bingham Farms, Michigan, is the one person who made a change in Arden's corporate culture within a very short period of time. Debra heard about Namaste Care, purchased the book, and started her own Namaste Care program a few days a week in the community studio. She happened to contact me just before I traveled to Michigan to lead a workshop. I invited her to attend, and the rest is history. After the workshop, Debra told me that one of her regional directors of operations as well as the director of lifestyle programs, Noreen Gray, had seen her program and they were both very impressed with what she was doing with Namaste Care. As luck would have it, I was going to Chicago that night, where they happened to be, and a dinner was arranged.

Two months later, Pauline, Noreen, and regional director of operations Margaret Reitmeyer spent the day visiting two established EPOCH Namaste Care programs in Massachusetts. That evening, we came up with a plan to implement Namaste Care in all of their communities. Within a week of our meeting I had approval to begin the first Arden Courts Namaste Care program in Winter Springs, Florida. Very shortly after this first program started, John Graham, vice president and general manager of the Assisted Living Division of HCR ManorCare, decided to make it the first national company to offer Namaste Care in all its assisted living communities.

For assisted living communities, Namaste Care completes the circle of activity programming for residents with dementia, from early to moderate and now advanced dementia. By adopting Namaste Care, Arden Courts raised the bar for the assisted living industry by providing at least 4 hours a day of programming 7 days a week for residents with advanced dementia. This chapter features my work with Arden Courts and several other companies.

## PARTICIPANT ASSESSMENT

In the United States there are fewer residents with advanced dementia in assisted living communities than in skilled nursing facilities.

In Arden Courts, approximately 20% of residents were advanced enough in their dementia that they could not participate in regular activity programs. Once the Namaste Care program opened, however, the number of residents who just enjoyed the peacefulness of the room grew. Many residents who wandered throughout the community were drawn to the room, and we quickly realized that we needed to have extra chairs for them. We placed comfortable chairs near the entrance to the room so residents can come and go without disrupting the program. Supplies such as blankets, combs, face cream, nail clippers, and emery boards are also available for the walk-ins. Dorothy was a resident whose story brings a smile to my face as I recall my first encounter with her.

## DOROTHY

Dorothy is a woman on the move. All day and sometimes into the evening, Dorothy wanders. This nonstop walking places her at risk of falling and losing weight, but usually no amount of coaxing can get her to sit for an activity. Dorothy is quite the social butterfly, flitting from one house to another. The day we introduced Namaste Care in her community, I was standing at the entrance to the living room that we had designated as the Namaste Care room, observing the program. Lovely music was playing; the scent of lavender filled the air. About eight residents were receiving hand massages and having their hair combed, engaged with a carer. Residents were tucked into their lounge chairs with soft, colorful blankets and looked happy and comfortable. I was delighted.

Then, Dorothy appeared at my side. She peered into the room and with a confused expression on her face said to me in a very loud voice, "Where did all these invalids come from?" I could see the peacefulness of Namaste Care disintegrating before me. Then I got creative and whispered to her, "This is a spa." She whispered back, "A spa?" and looked into the room again, this time with a smile. "Oh, a spa," she said knowingly. I then told her it was free and asked whether she wanted a hand massage. "Yes, please," she replied, and I led her to a chair by the window. One of the carers greeted her with a hug, tucked a blanket around her, and gave Dorothy her free hand massage. The next time I looked, Dorothy was asleep. She stayed in the "spa" for the entire morning, lowering her risk of falling and losing weight.

It seems that residents who walk around the community find the Namaste Care room a place to relax. Many of these same residents cannot find their own rooms, yet they manage to remember where and when Namaste Care takes place.

## PARTICIPANT SELECTION

The Arden Courts management team selects the first residents to participate in Namaste Care on the basis of their lack of participation or interest in the wide variety of activity programs each community offers on a daily basis. In all the assisted living communities in the United States, the United Kingdom, and Australia, we recommend that all staff receive information on the Namaste Care program before it begins. This ensures that everyone on the team understands what the program entails and how they can participate in it. Team members are also encouraged to suggest residents who they think could benefit from Namaste Care, because they are valued members of the team and have special relationships with the residents. Arden Courts has also developed a form that they will use on a regular basis to identify potential participants. This is an end-of-life program, and residents will not be in the program for long. When a resident dies or is discharged, another will be ready to take his or her place. There are usually more residents who could benefit from the program than can safely be accommodated in the room.

Residents who are receiving hospice services because of a diagnosis of advanced dementia are at the top of the list of participants; however, we had to teach team members and families that someone might be on hospice for another medical condition such as congestive heart failure and still participate in other activity programs, so he or she would not be suitable for Namaste Care. There has never been an instance when the team could not come up with enough residents to fill the Namaste Care room.

## SPACE

Assisted living communities are almost always more home-like than skilled nursing facilities because they adhere to a social model of care as opposed to a medical model. They are often smaller than the average 125-bed skilled nursing home, and many have just one floor with secured courtyards. In recent years, the assisted living industry has reacted to the growing population of residents with dementia by offering special dementia or memory care communities dedicated to caring for residents with some type of dementia. Many have "houses" or neighborhoods for a small group of residents within the footprint of the building. Arden Courts communities have been designed with a common center and four houses jutting out from each corner, with approximately 14 residents in each house. Residents can walk from one house to another, sit on each house's front porch, or attend programs in the studio or community center.

In the Arden Courts model, each community selects one house's living room to be the Namaste Care room. Some choose the house that has the most residents who would attend the program, others do the complete opposite. They think that the house with the higher-functioning residents attending programs in the central area community room will be quieter and more suited for Namaste Care. The room continues to be used as a living room when Namaste Care is not in session, so it is important to keep the home-like look of the room.

In larger assisted living communities, Namaste Care can find a home in an empty room or apartment. One program I helped with was in a large assisted living community that was home to residents without significant memory loss. They also had a secured dementia neighborhood. Residents could attend the program from anywhere in the community. When I use an apartment, I select one that is difficult to market, such as the one overlooking a graveyard; another had a view of the dumpster, both difficult to sell.

## DÉCOR

The décor in assisted living communities' common spaces is more home-like than the typical skilled nursing facility's day room. Living rooms in Arden Courts are furnished with love seats and comfortable chairs; however, to provide room for the four new reclining lounge chairs we needed for Namaste Care, and for the reclining wheelchairs used by some of the residents, we removed one love seat and a few chairs and tables. Wardrobes for storing blankets and an electric fireplace were purchased for the living room. Each community was given the freedom to decide the best way to make the room work for them. The residents who lived in that house were delighted that, when Namaste Care was not taking place, they had these comfortable chairs to use.

Geri-chairs used as recliners in nursing homes are not acceptable to use in the Arden Courts communities because they are institutional looking. In skilled facilities, this type of chair is commonly used for residents with advanced dementia. Under the Medicare hospice benefit, durable medical equipment related to the patient's diagnosis is provided, and comfortable chairs fall in that category. Hospice organizations are challenged to provide a suitable chair for patients, one that does not look institutional for an assisted living environment.

Like most large corporations, Arden Courts employed its own designers, who were very involved in choosing furniture and supplies for Namaste Care. I was very impressed when their designers, Holly Morgan and Susan Lancaster, flew to the first Arden Courts Namaste Care program in Winter Springs, Florida, so that they could understand the Namaste Care concept and select a recliner that met the residents' need for comfort and fit into the look of the living room. The reclining lounge chairs usually are the most expensive items that have to be purchased for Namaste Care. They must be fire rated and easy to clean. The design team also helped select the wardrobe for storing individual blankets and personal supplies. The pièce de résistance was the suggestion to purchase electric fireplaces that made the living room look and feel like home.

When I do not have the help of a corporate design team, I usually shop for sales and buy discounted chairs at furniture outlets. The maintenance department will know what to look for to meet fire regulations. As the assisted living population becomes more and more physically disabled, I believe that recliners will become a staple in living rooms.

In the large assisted living community I have already mentioned, we used an empty one-bedroom apartment for Namaste Care. We decorated it to look like a warm and inviting home by painting the off-white walls a pale peach color and hanging a wall-paper border of pastel flowers. Beige leather recliners were placed in the living room, and in what used to be the bedroom, lounge chairs faced a large flat-screen television.

With little money for this project, I found treasures in the storage area of the basement. Small tables and pictures that had been donated by families when their loved ones left the community were stored there, as were items used in model rooms; this basement became my bargain basement.

A small kitchenette in the apartment was perfect for the food and beverages used during the program. The food and beverage staff restocked it every day and made sure all the food handling and safety regulations were met. We made this small space look like a country kitchen with antique kitchen items placed on top of the cabinets and old-fashioned pictures of food products hung on the walls. A cookie jar placed on the counter, filled with easy-to-swallow treats, gave the kitchenette a welcoming look.

The bathroom was not used for toileting residents, but the sink was used to fill basins for hand and foot soaks and to clean supplies. A plastic shelving unit was set up in the shower and hidden behind a flowered shower curtain.

The maintenance department installed shelves in the closets for storage, and for a small amount of money we created a beautiful and private Namaste Care apartment. The room could be secured when it was not in use, so we were able to have real plants, and residents who were not memory impaired cared for them. As a matter of fact, the apartment was so beautiful, a prospective family member who saw it while touring the community agreed to move her mother in if she could have this apartment. So we moved everything to another apartment. Residents from the secured dementia neighborhood and residents from the traditional assisted living floors were transported to the apartment for the daily program.

## RESIDENT ROOMS

Like most assisted living communities, Arden Courts offers single rooms, as opposed to what is found in most skilled facilities, where two- or three-person rooms are not unusual. They also have their own toilets, and some have private showers; these features are not usually found in a skilled facility. Not having to worry about disturbing roommates makes it easier to bring Namaste Care in a rolling cart (see Chapter 5) to the bedside of a resident who is having difficulty sleeping or is agitated. Another benefit of having single rooms is that when a resident is actively dying, the family can have privacy. With single rooms, a community has no need for a Reagan Room, as they do in nursing facilities where private rooms are scarce. Jodi Woodside, executive director of Arden Courts in Winter Springs, Florida, relayed this story to me about the first resident to have the Namaste Care cart used when she was actively dying.

### OLIVIA

Olivia was the first resident for whom the Namaste Care traveling cart and the butterfly symbol on her door were used when she was actively dying. During Olivia's last days, a guitarist who had come to play for residents in the Community Center went to her room after he finished his performance. He sat by her bed and played songs that the staff told him were Olivia's favorites. Olivia had been unresponsive for several days, but as he played, tears flowed down her face and she held a carer's hand. She even moved her foot to the music. Her son was also a musician and had been playing for her almost every week because he knew that his mother loved music. As Olivia's dementia progressed and her son saw no response, he had stopped playing for her. During Olivia's last days our staff showed her husband and family how they could use some of the Namaste techniques, such as massaging her hands with lotion and gently combing her hair. Her family offered very positive feedback to us on the benefits of helping them become involved in the dying process in a very positive and personal way. As a result, one of the family members is now employed on our activity program staff.

## TEAM MEMBERS

Assisted living communities usually have fewer team members, especially nurses, who may not be in the community around the clock as they are in skilled nursing facilities. Carers are often in charge of the laundry, at least for residents' personal clothing. They also may have housekeeping tasks not assigned to nursing home carers. When we first proposed adding Namaste Care to the list of tasks they were responsible for, many carers thought this was something they could not add to their workload. However, as the program started, their resistance disappeared when they saw the amazing changes in residents. These are some of the comments from Arden Courts team members when we introduced Namaste Care.

> To be honest, in the beginning when we first heard about Namaste Care, everybody thought, "Oh no, something else I have to do," but once we saw what it was all about, everyone was on board 100%.
>
> One of the reasons I took this job in maintenance was to be part of caregiving, but over the years I am so busy with tasks I think I lost the reason why I was here. But seeing Namaste happen and spending time in the room with the residents, I know why I am here.

Because there are fewer team members in assisted living communities than in skilled nursing, the entire team has to help. A receptionist was a beautician before he came to Arden Courts. When he helps out in Namaste Care he styles the women's hair, and they love this extra pampering. When I saw his special talent and the reaction of the women, I thanked him as he left the room, and he replied, "No, thank you for this opportunity, the best part of my day."

Many management positions in skilled nursing are needed to meet regulations. Assisted living communities have fewer regulations and do not need as many people in management positions. For instance, most do not have a full-time education director, director of rehabilitation, or social worker. These roles are usually shared by the management staff in assisted living communities. Arden Courts calls this their "bench strength": Everyone does a bit of everything. It seems to me that this makes teamwork really work. More managers, especially nurses, are taking time to be part of the Namaste Care daily programming in Arden Courts communities than I have found in skilled facilities.

At Park Avenue, in a suburb of London, nurses are scheduled to be part of Namaste Care during the morning and afternoon sessions. I believe that increasing the nursing presence will result in a closer monitoring of changes in behaviors, and that will lead to decreasing use of antipsychotic medications. Nurses tell me that Namaste Care reminds them of why they became nurses in the first place. To my knowledge, nurses have not complained about the time they spend in the Namaste Care room.

## NAMASTE CARERS

Arden Courts has chosen to rotate carers in the Namaste Care room, following the current staffing model. Daily staff assignment sheets designate who will do Namaste Care. They are posted by the time clock for carers to see when they punch in for the shift. Each house has responsibility for the same time segment each day (e.g., Boathouse is responsible for the 10 to 10:30 A.M. slot each day). Carers are rotated to avoid burnout. Each house does 30 minutes so that they can still take care of the other residents who are not in the Namaste Care living room. The house that is scheduled to take the first half hour of Namaste Care is responsible for setting up the room, but the host house prepares the morning and afternoon beverages in cups with the residents' names on them. Each house has a dishwasher, so the cups can be washed after each session. Most skilled facilities use paper cups that are thrown away.

Each carer receives a list of residents he or she is assigned to care for and check on each hour. The carer also knows when the resident is scheduled for his or her 30 minutes in Namaste Care. This does not work unless the carers support each other, and when one is busy with a resident, other carers cover his or her shift. Many skilled facilities hire Namaste Carers, although some schedule their regular nursing assistants to rotate through the morning and afternoon programs.

One Arden Courts community initially scheduled just one carer for the 2-hour afternoon program but changed to the 30-minute assignments when all the carers told the resident service coordinator (nurse manager) they wanted some time in the program. Eventually, some carers may enjoy Namaste Care more than others and ask for a longer assignment. One of the strengths I have observed in Arden Courts is that the managers listen to the carers and make changes as requested.

## ROUND-THE-CLOCK NURSING

Arden Courts has scheduled round-the-clock nursing to meet the increasingly challenging medical needs of their residents as they "age in place." Nurses will be available to monitor residents' medical needs throughout the progression of dementia. Having a nurse available may also help to decrease hospitalizations. Hospitalizing residents with advanced dementia is often more burdensome than beneficial, and the costs of even one day of a hospital stay are causing a tremendous drain on health care resources in the United States.

## LIFE STORIES

Social histories are mandated for skilled nursing facilities, whereas assisted living communities can decide what information they need to gather before a resident moves in. They do not have social workers, so gathering this information is a shared responsibility of the management team. Arden Courts asks families to complete a Resident Lifestyle Biography before the resident moves into the community. They developed another form called the Namaste Care Story. The form reads, "Everyone has a story to tell! Building Namaste Friendships Piece by Piece." A staff member completes this form by talking to family members and the carers who have the most up-to-date information on food preferences and the resident's routine. The back of the form is used for updates, such as where the resident prefers to sit and the foods he or she enjoys as part of Namaste Care. The completed Namaste Care Story is placed in a binder with a picture of the resident on the front and pictures of the resident's past. Some high schools have a community service requirement for graduation. This would be a perfect project for such students; they can read the residents' histories and print pictures from the Internet of where they lived or schools they attended. One resident had pictures of advertisements for old Broadway musicals. The family told the carers that the resident loved going to New York and attended many Broadway shows. Another could speak only Polish and was a devout Catholic. Her binder contained the Lord's Prayer in Polish, which she would read each day. This way of communicating the resident's past history and present preferences gives carers and volunteers in Namaste Care the information they need to get to know residents who may not be verbal at this time of life. Some residents enjoy looking at the pictures from their past.

### CHARLES

> Charles was a well-educated man from a small African country. He knew several languages, but as his dementia progressed he could speak only his native language, and no one understood what he was saying. He was taken to the Namaste Care room and settled in a lounge chair. A large picture of him with his wife and four children was placed on a table in front of him. He looked around the room for quite a while, absorbing the calm atmosphere. All of a sudden he took the picture in both hands and with a broad smile said in English, "This is my beautiful family!"

The binders created in Arden Courts are good examples of the correct way to share social histories (life stories) with everyone. I have always objected to the practice of hiding them in charts, as skilled facilities do.

## EARLY-ONSET DEMENTIA

In the past few years, the number of people with early-onset dementia (occurring before the age of 65) has increased. Arden Courts communities are seeing more people in their 40s and 50s moving into a heartbreaking situation for their spouses and young families. Although studies do not support my observation that the dementia progresses faster in this younger population, most of the health care professionals I ask feel the same way. One woman I will never forget is Desiree.

### DESIREE

> I met Desiree a few years ago and was struck by her youth and beauty. She was only 62 years old and was a very distressed resident who constantly walked slowly around the neighborhood, crying. The staff did everything they could to comfort her, a psychologist was of no help, and none of the antidepressants were helpful. One day while I was visit-

ing, a carer brought Desiree to the Namaste Care room and sat next to her, running her fingers through Desiree's hair and telling her how much she was loved and how beautiful she was. Desiree fell into a peaceful sleep with a beautiful smile on her face. When she woke, I was sitting across from her, and she looked at me and said, "I love you," to which I replied, "I love you too." She left the room and continued walking around the neighborhood, but she was smiling, and she told everyone she met that she loved them. She often wandered into the Namaste Care room and always fell asleep in this comforting space.

She has been a resident for 3 years and is in the terminal stage of her disease. Desiree is now a hospice patient and in a reclining wheelchair. She is not able to make eye contact and has no verbal skills left. As I reflect on my memories of Desiree, I realize how Namaste Care has provided quality of life for her throughout her time in this community. Whereas once she was sad and wandering around the neighborhood, she is now peacefully sleeping in the Namaste Care room, surrounded by love. I said my goodbyes to her as I left the community because I believe she will not be there for my next visit.

Helping younger residents feel at home with a mostly geriatric population is a challenge. One executive director told me that he has a younger resident who feels as if he is a volunteer and does not see himself as part of a community of so many "old people." They have given him a name tag that designates him as a volunteer, and staff ask for his help, keeping him busy and helping him feel as if he can still contribute to the community. The executive director plans to try him as a volunteer in the Namaste Care room, helping carers gather supplies or just holding residents' hands.

Another community has several residents who are former nurses and work as volunteers in the Namaste Care room. They are delightfully happy caring for patients again. There is always a staff person in the room, so these volunteers will not be in a situation that places them or any resident in an unsafe position.

## MEDICAL DIRECTORS

Skilled nursing facilities are required by law to employ a medical director; assisted living communities in some states are not. Arden

Courts employ what they call advisory physicians communities. One of the goals of Namaste Care is to reduce or eliminate the use of antipsychotics, and some physicians are reluctant to do this if a resident is not having problems with the medication. Medical directors can be helpful in speaking to other physicians about reducing medications. They are also helpful in speaking to families about end-of-life medical interventions such as hospitalization, cardiopulmonary resuscitation, and tube feeding. The goal of Namaste Care is for residents to have a calm, peaceful death in their own rooms, in a community where the carers know and love them.

## SALES AND MARKETING

Arden Courts believes that the addition of Namaste Care will provide a new program of meaningful activities for their residents who have aged in place and are now in the advanced stage of dementia. They have elected to market Namaste Care as an integral program that rounds out their other structured programs. With the addition of Namaste Care, Arden Courts now embraces early, middle, and advanced dementia in their communities.

These residents are always well groomed and often found asleep in front of the television or isolated in their rooms because they can no longer participate in activity programs. When prospective residents' families tour the facility, the sight of people slumped over in their wheelchairs is not the impression any community wants to convey. As sales and marketing people like to say, "You never get a second chance to make a first impression." With residents comfortably seated in the Namaste Care room and most other residents attending activity programs, almost every resident is engaged and happy.

Some families who tour assisted living communities are shown the daily schedule of activity programs but feel that their family member would not participate in any activity, so this has no benefit for them. When they are shown Namaste Care, they feel that this unique program may appeal to their loved one, and as one marketing person said to me, "This sometimes clinches a sale."

An assisted living community that needs to increase its census might decide to implement Namaste Care to give their marketers something new to talk about with referral sources. Even when families are looking for a home for someone in an earlier stage of dementia, they may appreciate knowing that the community provides programming for all levels of dementia.

As programs open, the wise marketing staff will schedule a grand opening complete with a ribbon-cutting ceremony, with a story and pictures that can be submitted to the local paper. Mary Hayes, program service coordinator of Arden Courts of Winter Springs, Florida, had her residents with early memory loss make lavender sachets for referral sources, and she also gathered her "cooks" (the residents) to make lavender cookies for a marketing event.

Marketing materials describing Namaste Care should be developed and information on the program added to the company's Web site. My only request to anyone naming their program *Namaste Care* is that they meet the standards I have established. Reputations are ruined when a community promises a service that has no integrity.

## OUTCOMES

The outcomes of Namaste Care in assisted living are similar to those we have found in skilled nursing. Families visit more often and feel the visits are more enjoyable. With greater intake of beverages, nursing staff report fewer skin tears and fewer urinary tract infections. Falls also decrease. Use of medication to treat depression or anxiety may be discontinued. And team members in skilled facilities report that they feel their own spirits lift when Namaste Care is offered to residents who can no longer benefit from other activities.

Families are very pleased when they see their loved ones in the program. Executive director Jodi Woodside of Arden Courts of Winter Springs, Florida, sent me this comment about feedback they have received from families since initiating Namaste Care:

> Family involvement was a great surprise. Some family members find it easier to visit during Namaste. They now have something to do with the resident in a loving, calm environment. It has taken the pressure off of them. They no longer need to figure out what to do or what to talk about during the visit.

Several families have said they felt that the last days and months of their loved one's life were made special by Namaste Care. One letter from the daughter of a resident said, "I feel a special gratitude that Mom was included in your Namaste program and that your nurturing brought brightness to her everyday life there."

## THE NAMASTE CARE HOUSE

Arden Courts recognized that keeping residents within their community when they reach the advanced stage of dementia requires more carers. In 2012, they opened the first dedicated Namaste Care house in Arden Courts of Chagrin Falls, Ohio, as a pilot project. All other Arden Courts communities will continue to offer 4 hours a day of Namaste Care programming while the success of the Namaste Care house is evaluated. The house they selected, Garden Path, has one additional carer for each of the three shifts. Although the monthly fee is higher, families are delighted that they do not have to move their loved one to a nursing facility to receive the extra physical care they need.

Each of the four houses in an Arden Courts community has the same layout, so re-creating a resident's room in the Namaste Care house is relatively easy; most residents do not even realize they have been moved. In addition to the four hours devoted to the Namaste Care daily program, team members bake bread and cookies to create tantalizing aromas that stimulate appetites. Special activities are offered throughout the day. Executive Director Erin Pfenning has seen positive changes in residents, including one that occurred on the first day that the Namaste Care program was offered.

### ROSE

Rose is a female resident in the advanced stage of dementia. She also has very poor eyesight and spatial difficulties. She typically spends her days calling out for her husband or pleading to go home. Often, to the dismay of carers and her family, Rose will say "I want to die." On a "good day," Rose listens to music on the front porch of her "house."

The peaceful feeling that fills the Namaste Care house gave Erin hope that taking Rose to the daily program would improve her quality of life. Rose was taken to the Namaste Care program room in a wheelchair and transferred to a comfortable lounge chair. Although Rose was at first somewhat resistive to this, Erin felt that the combination of music that she knew Rose enjoyed and the tranquility of the room might calm her. "I watched as the stiffness and worry left her body," Erin said. "I made her comfortable with a few small pillows and a soft fluffy blanket. Rose started to talk in a quiet voice and even laughed a little as I was gently washing and moisturizing her face and brushing her hair. In this brief period of time, Rose became animated and acted as if her dementia had disappeared. When I asked her if she was enjoying herself, she said 'This is the best day of my life.' This happened on the first day of Namaste Care, and Rose was the first person in the program. What a great start!"

Since that day positive changes have occurred in many of the residents who live in the new Namaste Care house. Carers are excited to know that they are making a difference in the residents' lives. Erin reports that every day she walks into the Namaste Care house, carers have another amazing story to tell her.

Families have also been thrilled to see their loved ones smiling and being responsive to their surroundings and the activities offered to them. They remark that their visits are longer and they feel less frustrated because the carers can tell them what their loved one enjoys. Family members can be seen giving hand massages or offering bits of a favorite ice cream to their loved one. It has been a pleasant surprise to see how quickly the Namaste Care house has become a Namaste Care home.

# CHAPTER 8

# Quality of Life at the End of Life

There is no profit in curing the body
if in the process we destroy the soul.

CITY OF HOPE, credo (Comprehensive Cancer Center)

Namaste Care™ is for people whose dementia has advanced to a point where physicians are talking to their families about a palliative approach to care. This means that the focus of care is on comfort and relief from distress rather than on curative medical treatment. Ideally, the family and the patient have already discussed some of the end-of-life decisions they may face, but often this is not the case.

From the time their loved one begins to show signs of dementia, family members are faced with a multitude of medical and psychosocial decisions that become more complex as the disease progresses. For many families, especially couples, the possible diagnosis of Alzheimer's disease is too frightening to face, so they ignore or rationalize the signs of dementia. Most seniors are well aware that no cure exists. Even in cases of irreversible dementia, some families choose not to tell their loved one. However, this denies the person with dementia the opportunity to make decisions about care, including end-of-life care, at a point when he or she is still able to make decisions. Making decisions about one's own fate—to whatever degree is possible—is every person's right, as is the right to know one's medical condition.

## DIFFICULT DECISIONS

People in the early stages of dementia can make decisions about finances, designate a power of attorney (POA), and participate in writing advance directives and living wills. The family and physician should initiate discussions about potential medical decisions as soon as the diagnosis is made. When the person with dementia is involved in planning for end-of-life care, some of the burden family members feel as the disease progresses is lifted. Most importantly, taking these legal steps will help ensure that their loved one's wishes will be honored.

To participate meaningfully in any of these decisions, a person must first be aware of the diagnosis of dementia. Virginia Bell and David Troxel, who developed the Best Friends approach to Alzheimer's care, created a "Dementia Bill of Rights" (see Appendix E). The first right is "To be informed of one's diagnosis." When the person does not want to hear or face the news, he or she usually just ignores it; most want to know.

The following situation occurred in a nursing facility and shows how adaptable residents are to receiving the diagnosis of Alzheimer's disease.

### MICHAEL

Michael had been having problems with memory for several years. When he became lost while driving home, his family took him to a physician, who, after conducting a series of tests, diagnosed Michael with probable Alzheimer's disease. His family refused to allow the doctor to tell Michael what was wrong with him for fear he would become depressed. When he fell and broke his hip, the family decided he was no longer safe at home and admitted him to a nursing facility. He was also having trouble remembering names, even those of his grandchildren.

Michael was becoming more and more distressed because he did not know what was happening to him. He kept asking the social worker what was wrong with him and then forgetting that he had asked, so he returned to her office to ask her again and again and again. She was not authorized to disclose his diagnosis. Eventually, she scheduled a meeting with the family members to discuss their father's right to know about the diagnosis. They reluctantly agreed to let him speak with his physician. A private meeting was set up in the social worker's office. When the physician explained that he believed Michael was in the beginning stage of Alzheimer's disease, Michael replied, "Thank God. I thought I was going crazy. I can handle Alzheimer's disease; after all, President Reagan did."

## FAMILY DECISION MAKING

Decision making is a process. In the early stages of dementia, the goal may be to prolong life; during the middle stage the goals shift to maintaining function; and as the disease reaches the end stages, the goal of care is to provide comfort using a palliative approach to care (Volicer, 2012). The social worker in the nursing facility should begin discussions with family members, and whenever possible with the resident, as soon as the person is moved into the facility. In the United Kingdom and Australia, social work services are available in the local community if needed, but for the most part it is the care home managers who schedule family meetings.

In the early stage of a dementing illness, the resident may be able to make end-of-life decisions. Unfortunately, by the time many residents are admitted to a nursing facility, they are usually unable to participate in these discussions because they can no longer comprehend the issues.

Ideally, when a resident is admitted to a nursing facility, a POA has been designated and a living will is in place or the responsible party is clear about the resident's wishes. However, many residents and their family members have not had conversations about end-of-life decisions and may still be in denial that Alzheimer's disease is a terminal illness. In that case, decisions will continue to be made informally, without legal sanction, by the family and physician. It is helpful to have ongoing family meetings so that decisions do not have to be made at the time of a crisis. When nursing and team members determine that Namaste Care is appropriate for a resident, it is an opportunity to make sure that the family recognizes that their loved one has reached the advanced stage of the disease. And if end-of-life planning has not already been discussed and agreed upon, this is an ideal time to encourage families to look ahead and make plans for a peaceful and dignified death. Without these plans, the resident may be subjected to cardiopulmonary resuscitation (CPR), tube feeding, and hospitalization, all of which are more burdensome than beneficial to residents with advanced dementia. A better "treatment" at this stage of the disease is the daily Namaste Care program, which provides comfort and reassurance to families that their loved one is receiving a form of care that promotes quality of life at the end of life.

Unfortunately, problems can and do emerge when the family has no advance directives to follow and the family members disagree on medical decisions. The death in 2005 of Terri Schiavo, a young Florida woman who was comatose and did not leave written advance directives, threw the United States into a fierce debate over end-of-life decisions. This emotionally charged case went to the floor of the Senate and eventually to the Supreme Court. The public battle pitted Terri's husband and parents against each other in the bright spotlight of the media. If advance directives or a living will had been written, this battle would not have occurred. On a positive note, as a result of this case, more Americans now have signed living wills than at any other point in history.

## LEGAL ACTIONS FOR END-OF-LIFE CARE

There are a number of ways in which a person can communicate his or her health care and end-of-life wishes; some are legal, others are more informal, such as conversations that take place before memory loss makes decision making impossible. The most common ways to make and share end-of-life decisions are discussed in this section. It should be repeated that Namaste Care is not a form of medical treatment; it is usually considered an activity program that does not require family consent.

## Advance Directives

Advance directives can be either written or oral. Written advance directives are sometimes called living wills. Advance directives specify which medical interventions the person would like to receive or avoid. However, it is very difficult to anticipate and specify which medical interventions might be needed, so advance directives are often very general and may not be useful in the case of dementia. What is more useful is the appointment of someone to have power of attorney for medical decisions. This person should know the wishes of the person with dementia before he or she can no longer make medical decisions for himself or herself.

## Power of Attorney for Medical Decisions

Each state determines the procedures for declaring a person legally incompetent. A person must be declared incompetent by a court of law, which will also appoint a POA. This is sometimes a long and expensive process. Until a POA is appointed, the resident is legally in charge of his or her own decisions—an unrealistic task for people with advanced dementia. If no POA is appointed, most states have a law that determines which relative is the designated proxy. Despite the designation of a POA or designated proxy, disagreements can still occasionally arise between family members with regard to care and treatment decisions. Facility team members sometimes feel caught in the middle.

## Physician Orders for Life-Sustaining Treatment

The Physician Orders for Life-Sustaining Treatment (POLST) program is designed to improve the quality of care people receive at the end of life and to respect the wishes of people with an advanced illness (see http://www.ohsu.edu/polst/programs/index.htm). The POLST form is different from an advance directive because it is a physician order for specific treatment limitations. It is based on effective communication of patient wishes, documentation of medical orders on a brightly colored form, and a promise by health care professionals to honor these wishes. It was developed in 1990 as a quality initiative to improve patient care and to reduce medical errors by creating a system that identifies and respects patients' wishes for medical treatment throughout all health care settings. The system focuses on a growing segment of the U.S. population, those with advanced chronic progressive illness, and it elicits, communicates, and honors their wishes through portable medical orders. The majority of states either have some type of POLST program or are in the process of approving one. The form has been modified to allow for proxy advanced care planning for people with dementia (Volicer et al., 2002).

## The Federal Patient Self-Determination Act

The purpose of the Patient Self-Determination Act (PSDA, P.L. 101-508, 1990) was to inform patients of their rights regarding decisions about their own medical care and to ensure that these rights are communicated by health care providers. Specifically, the rights ensured are those of patients to dictate their future care (by means such as living will or power of attorney), should they become incapacitated (http://www.americanbar.org/groups/public_education/resources/law_issues_for_consumers/patient_self_determination_act.html). This act requires nursing facilities that participate in Medicare or Medicaid programs to provide residents and their families with written policies on advance directives. On admission, residents and their families are given copies of these policies and must sign a statement indicating that they received them. Each person's medical record must include information on the resident's advance directives, if they exist. Namaste Care nursing and social work staff members can help family members make difficult decisions by providing education on the burdens and benefits of medical interventions.

Planning for end-of-life care can be overwhelming for families, but there are resources readily available. Searching the Internet will yield numerous Web sites that provide guidance on drafting living wills, which must be specifically designed for individual states, as well as sample forms.

All states have some type of ombudsman program, which provides advocates for people living in residential long-term care settings and can help residents and families with a variety of issues, including referring families to organizations that offer legal assistance. If a resident is eligible for hospice care, hospice staff will provide counseling to families regarding end-of-life decision making. Hospice also offers grief and bereavement services for up to a year after the death.

### Gold Standard Framework

In the United Kingdom, the Gold Standard Framework (GSF, http://www.goldstandardsframework.org.uk) for care homes is a program that enables care homes and other health care settings to provide high-quality care for all residents nearing the end of life. It helps physicians and team members identify residents who are in the last years of life, assess their needs, symptoms, and preferences, and develop a plan of care, enabling residents to die in a manner that honors their wishes.

## MEDICAL DECISIONS

The following information, drawn from studies of nursing facility residents with advanced dementia, supports the primary goal of Namaste Care philosophy to provide comfort care.

### Cardiopulmonary Resuscitation

Initiating CPR on a resident with advanced dementia is burdensome and rarely successful. The numerous complications of this treatment include fractured ribs, admission to a hospital's intensive care unit (ICU), and placement on a mechanical respirator (Volicer, 2012). The ICU is especially frightening to those with dementia, and most people admitted to the ICU will need to be sedated. Studies show that of 114 nursing facility residents who were admitted to a hospital after CPR, only 10% were discharged; the rest died in the hospital (Ghusan, Teasdale, Pepe, & Ginger, 1995).

### Hospitalization

Hospitalizing a nursing facility resident with advanced dementia is ill advised. Unless the resident absolutely cannot be treated comfortably in the nursing facility, a transfer to an acute care center often results in a decline in the ability to transfer, increased risk of decubitus ulcers, and weight loss (Volicer, McKee, & Hewitt, 2001). Many residents who are hospitalized return to the nursing facility with indwelling catheters and on significantly more medications.

From the moment the ambulance crew arrives, the nursing facility resident with advanced dementia is plunged into a world that is alien and terrifying. Upon arrival at the hospital, the resident usually spends time in the emergency room. A variety of tests, confusing and occasionally painful, terrify the resident who cannot comprehend the reason for these procedures. More often than not, the resident is then transported back to the facility. If the resident is admitted to the hospital, anxiety intensifies.

Acute care staff members are not as familiar with the needs of patients with advanced dementia as nursing facility staff are. People with advanced dementia are unable to understand that they cannot get out of bed without assistance and do not comprehend the purpose of items such as catheters and intravenous (IV) tubes; many times, they must be restrained or sedated in order to keep these interventions in place. Pressure ulcers are a danger for frail residents who are restrained in their beds for long periods of time. Residents with advanced dementia need to be hand fed and coaxed into eating, a time-consuming task for nurses. They also need to be offered liquid several times per day because they are not able to pour and drink.

Many residents return from the hospital with more medications. In order to manage confused or distressed behavior, the hospital may have placed the resident on antipsychotics or benzodiazepines, sometimes both. The resident may also be given medication to aid sleeping. All of these medications can produce dry mouth, constipation, and lethargy, among other unpleasant conditions.

Once in the acute care setting, residents experience unpleasant medical interventions such as blood tests, X-rays, and computed tomography scans. When considering whether to hospitalize a resident, one must weigh the burdens and benefits of these procedures. Will the resident's life be more comfortable as a result of the hospitalization? It is important to remember, and to remind families, that decisions can be changed at any time. For example, if a resident breaks her hip, her family must decide whether to surgically repair the hip of the resident who has not walked for some time and probably will not walk again. In this case, consider the fact that the hip may heal on its own with bed rest and appropriate pain medication. The resident may rest comfortably in her own familiar bed or in a reclining chair in the Namaste Care room among staff members who understand her needs.

## Tube Feeding

In the United States, decisions about tube feeding seem to be emotionally charged. The pros and cons of this procedure must be considered before a feeding tube is inserted. There is evidence that feeding with a nasogastric (NG) tube or through a percutaneous endoscopic gastrostomy (PEG) tube does not increase survival rates of people with advanced dementia. Research also indicates that tube feeding does not prevent aspiration pneumonia and may actually increase its risk (Finucane, Christmas, & Travis, 1999). The belief that tube feeding will lower the risk of pressure ulcers and decrease the risk of infection has been disproved in studies. The procedure to insert a feeding tube is uncomfortable and can be expensive.

An NG tube can be inserted by a nurse. Because NG tubes are uncomfortable, residents are often restrained or have mitts placed on their hands so they will not pull out the tube. In a study of patients who were alert and oriented and who had recovered from a stay in the ICU, results showed that tube feeding was the most uncomfortable procedure that the patients encountered, more uncomfortable than being attached to a ventilator. Being restrained was third on the list of uncomfortable procedures (Morrison et al., 1998).

A PEG tube must be inserted by a specialty physician and requires hospitalization. Evaluation for a PEG tube insertion requires consultation with a speech therapist to document that food is not entering the lungs, as well as the services of an X-ray technician and radiologist to determine swallowing capabilities. This test requires swallowing barium, something the resident with advanced dementia may not be able to do. Inserting PEG tubes is a surgical operation requiring anesthetic. As with any surgery, there are risks inherent in the procedure, including infection and increased confusion from the anesthetic.

Antidepressant medications might be an alternative to tube feeding for residents who can still swallow but have stopped eating. Refusal of food may also be a conscious wish of a resident who can no longer communicate verbally (Volicer, 2012). We honor our residents by not forcing them to eat or drink; however, most residents can be tempted with beverages and small amounts of preferred food, such as orange slices, chocolate, and lollipops, until they begin to actively die. The enjoyment of food may be one of the last pleasures that residents with advanced dementia have.

The following story about Nathan and his mother, Julia, is one example of how a son was able to feel comfortable about keeping his mother in the nursing facility rather than hospitalizing her for hydration therapy.

## JULIA

Nathan was recently divorced and retired and had little to do except focus on caring for his mother, Julia. He visited every day. Clearly, he was devoted to her and was stricken with grief that she was in the last stage of dementia. Julia slept most of the time, and getting her to eat or drink anything was a miracle. During his visits, usually at lunch, Nathan would become either elated that she ate or drank something or very frustrated when she refused all attempts to feed her. He often had her hospitalized for hydration therapy when she refused to eat and drink. Nathan told me that he felt he had to do something; he could not let his mother starve. His mother's physician discouraged him from having a tube inserted but did agree to hospitalize her for hydration therapy.

The day Namaste Care began, Julia was sleeping in her wheelchair. When I approached her to say hello, I observed black-and-blue marks all over her arms. Alarmed, I was informed by the staff that Julia had once again spent a few days in the hospital for IV therapy. The places where the needles had been inserted and where the restraints had been secured were bruised. Julia pulled out the IV without the restraints, but her skin was fragile and tore easily. Even a small amount of pressure could cause skin discoloration and abrasions. It was heartbreaking to see this tiny woman looking as if she had been in a prize fight and lost.

Julia was transported to the Namaste Care room and moved from her wheelchair into a reclining lounge chair, and a soft quilt was tucked around her. Small pillows were positioned under her arms, and a lollipop was offered to her. She opened her eyes and smiled when she tasted the sweetness, and she sucked greedily on it. We had our first success story. Her son arrived shortly after the room opened and panicked when he could not find his mother in her usual place in the day room. The staff led him to the Namaste Care room, where soft music was playing, the scent of lavender was in the air, and his mother, very comfortable in the lounge chair, was sucking on her lollipop, eyes opened and twinkling with delight.

Nathan started to cry. I panicked. What had we done wrong? He said it had been so long since he had seen his mother so happy and comfortable. He began to tell me how awful he felt seeing his mother in the hospital, about the ambulance ride, painful testing, and the restraints needed to keep his mother from pulling out the IV. We talked about how difficult it was for him to let go of his mother. He asked whether she could be in Namaste Care every day. When told yes, he went to the nurse's station and informed them not to hospitalize her any more. He could see how comfortable his mother was and wanted her to stay with the staff who knew and loved her. She died a few weeks later, and Nathan said that he was at peace knowing that her last days were spent in the arms of the Namaste Carer.

## Treatment of Infections

Every nursing facility has infection control procedures that must be followed. Infections are the most common complication for people with advanced dementia. Respiratory infections and urinary tract infections are the most common of these. Although infections are routinely treated in the early stages of the disease, when the person still has years of high-quality life ahead, at some point in the advanced stage of the disease the family and physician should discuss whether antibiotics should still be used. If comfort is the main concern, then over-the-counter fever medication and morphine may be the treatments of choice.

Pneumonia is a common infection. Studies reveal that the residents with advanced dementia who are treated in the nursing facility are as likely to survive the episode as those who are treated in the hospital (Fried, Gillick, & Lipsitz, 1995). Urinary tract infections can be also treated with comfort measures in the nursing facility.

Residents with advanced dementia are unable to report early symptoms and sometimes do not run a fever, one of the easiest ways to identify infections. By the time they do show signs of infection, its severity can make curing it difficult. If antibiotics are to be used, a diagnostic work-up is needed. This could involve blood tests, X-rays, catheterization, or other uncomfortable procedures.

All these diagnostic procedures should be explained to the family members so that they can make an informed decision. Antibiotics also have side effects such as nausea and diarrhea (including *Clostridium difficile* infections) that would decrease the resident's comfort. Many times, the resident can be made comfortable without antibiotics, and the simplest treatment may be the best.

## JAMES

> James was clearly in the advanced stage of dementia. He had almost stopped eating and drinking. He weighed less than 100 pounds. All of his needs were being met by staff; he was unable to speak, needed total care for his activities of daily living, was nonambulatory, and could be out of bed only for short periods of time because he was at high risk for skin breakdown. He began to show signs of a respiratory illness, probably pneumonia, the nurses thought. The physician ordered X-rays, and James was treated with antibiotics and given an oxygen mask. Despite his frailty, James made it very clear that he did not want the mask on his face. His small hands pulled and tugged at it until he was able to get it off. James was definitely communicating his discomfort. The Namaste Care nurse assessed his behavior and evaluated the effectiveness of the uncomfortable mask. The physician agreed that comfort was the goal and discontinued the order for oxygen. James went back to bed and went peacefully to sleep. He survived pneumonia on his terms.

Team members are always listening to and watching residents who communicate with body language when verbal communication is no longer possible, and they share their observations during meetings and in the resident's interdisciplinary care plan.

## Care Plans

In all countries where I have worked or spoken about Namaste Care, some form of care planning is part of the services they offer. The interdisciplinary care team can schedule care plan meetings to help make families aware of the potential medical issues that are associated with Alzheimer's disease and other dementias and to help them make decisions about the goals of care. These goals of care change as dementia progresses. Hospitalization might be avoided, for instance, in the middle stage, as the goal of care is to maintain function. In the advanced stage of dementia, however, the goal is comfort and the burdens associated with hospitalization usually outweigh the benefits.

Care plan meetings are held on a regular basis according to federal and state regulations and whenever a significant change of condition is noted. The facility must inform family members of the date and time of the conference and place a copy of the letter in the resident's medical record. If the family does not attend the meeting, someone on the care planning team should call the family to discuss the care plan or be sure to review the plan during the family's visits.

Namaste Care team members should attempt to involve as many family members as possible in the discussion of the care plan and goals of care so that the family understands and supports the interdisciplinary team. Some options for getting families to meetings include the following:

- Schedule meetings when the majority of family members can attend.

- Involve family members who are unable to come to the facility by using telephone or Internet conference calling.

- Be flexible enough to schedule a meeting on the weekend if that is the only time the majority of family members can attend.

- Use e-mail to connect with family members, making sure that privacy regulations are met.

Meetings with families help to build strong connections with department managers and team members. It is important to schedule enough time for the meetings so that family members can talk about their feelings and so that team members can discuss decisions that may have to be made in the future. This will give the family time to consider the various treatment issues.

## Nursing Procedures

Good nursing practice and nursing facility regulations require certain nursing tasks such as weighing residents, monitoring blood pressure readings, taking temperatures, and measuring pulse and respiration rates. However, some of these procedures may be changed for the comfort of the resident with advanced dementia. Under physician orders and federal and state regulations, the number of times these tasks are done may be changed. Taking weights, for instance, may be unnecessary when the family and physician decide not to use tube feeding or any other intervention when a resident is refusing food. Instead, the resident's upper arm or thigh could be measured, a more comfortable procedure than weighing. If the physician and family decide to change routine nursing procedures, the resident's care plan must be changed.

## Medication

Medications may have unpleasant side effects. At a certain point in the life of a resident with advanced dementia, medication for chronic conditions may be discontinued. Vitamins and medications for lowering cholesterol levels or for slowing the progression of Alzheimer's disease have limited effectiveness and are not indicated at this time unless they are used for the resident's comfort. Medications that alleviate joint pain or discomfort from arthritis and other medications used for the comfort of the resident are always indicated.

## PALLIATIVE CARE

Decisions about care options for nursing facility residents are made throughout the disease process. When a palliative or comfort care approach is used, it sometimes appears that care is being decreased.

Palliative care is often confused with hospice care, and families feel as if it means their loved one will die soon. It is important for physicians, nursing staff, and social workers to explain to families that palliative care relieves and prevents the suffering of residents while trying to increase the quality of their lives. Unlike hospice care, which focuses on the last 6 months of life, palliative care is appropriate for patients in all disease stages.

Palliative care is defined as "whole person care for patients whose diseases are not responsive to curative treatments" (Maxwell, et al., 2008). The goal of palliative care is "to prevent and relieve suffering and to support the best possible quality of life for patients and the families regardless of the stage of the disease" (National Consensus Project, 2009).

Namaste Care shows families that their loved ones are receiving more specialized services and more activities that are meaningful at this stage of their lives. Quality of life is the focus. The emphasis is not on the number of days left in a person's life but on the quality of those days. Namaste Care honors each resident, surrounding him or her with a loving environment and in the presence of others.

One of the primary goals of Namaste Care is to provide comfort in all aspects of life for residents with advanced dementia. The term *comfort care* usually means not using aggressive medical interventions such as hospitalization, tube feeding, blood tests, and other uncomfortable or confusing diagnostic procedures. Namaste Care believes that palliative care measures include the following:

- Managing pain and discomfort so that each resident is comfortable at all times
- Offering activities of daily living (ADLs), which include dressing, grooming, oral care, toileting, feeding, bathing, and ambulation, as meaningful activities
- Clothing residents for comfort
- Providing a comfortable environment

## PAIN

Alzheimer's disease and other dementias do not cause physical pain, yet many residents with dementia experience untreated pain from other medical conditions such as cancer, fractures, arthritis, tooth decay, and osteoporosis. Pain is often undertreated or not treated at all because residents with advanced dementia cannot report the pain (Williams, Zimmerman, Sloane, & Reed, 2005). Undiagnosed pain occurs in 26%–83% of nursing facility residents and is a significant problem (Huffman & Kunik, 2000). Residents with dementia depend on staff to recognize when they are in pain and to provide relief. Therefore, residents must be continually evaluated for pain and discomfort by the Namaste Care team.

Namaste Care partners and nurses usually are the first to recognize discomfort; however, all team members are expected to report behaviors that may be signs of pain. Namaste Carers often are the first to notice such changes in residents because they see them every day for a significant number of hours, more than any other team member.

Namaste Care incorporates the hospice philosophy regarding pain: Believe the resident. If the resident is able to communicate and says or acts as if he or she is in pain, then the resident is treated and monitored to make sure the medication has been successful. Without adequate pain management, residents in pain cannot experience improved quality of life. Any attempt by the Namaste Carer to provide meaningful activities will be difficult or impossible. In order to maintain quality of life, recognizing, assessing, treating, and monitoring pain in residents with advanced dementia is crucial.

Determining the level and location of pain in a resident with advanced dementia is like solving a puzzle, and nurses and care partners must uncover the clues. Residents may show the following nonverbal signs of pain:

- Facial expressions that show discomfort, such as grimaces, frown lines, and tense expressions
- Tension in the body, stiffness, or unwillingness to respond to a request to move

- Decreased ability to assist in performing ADLs
- Noisy, labored, or rapid breathing
- Shrinking or wincing when touched
- Rubbing a part of the body
- Avoiding the use of a part of the body
- Curling into a fetal position
- Decreased range of motion
- Keeping eyes closed

Vocal signs of pain include the following:

- Saying, "It hurts"
- Saying, "No!"
- Screaming
- Swearing
- Moaning
- Crying or whimpering
- Changing vocalization or tone
- Making repetitive sounds

A resident in pain may exhibit the following behaviors:

- Resist transferring from bed to a chair
- Fight attempts of staff to perform ADLs
- Grab staff
- Refuse to eat
- Appear restless
- Act agitated
- Refuse to engage in preferred activities
- Have problems sleeping
- Show anxiety
- Exhibit mood changes

Care partners usually are the first ones to notice signs of discomfort or pain when they are dressing or changing the residents. They must immediately notify a nurse, who can assess the level or intensity of the pain, the location, and the potential cause. Pain assessment is necessary to determine the appropriate treatment.

## Assessment of Pain

Pain can be acute or chronic. Acute pain is usually temporary; such as the pain associated with dental problems or a skin tear. Acute pain will cause the resident to cry out, moan, or have pained facial expressions. This type of pain can be treated with any number of pain medications and usually resolves quickly. The symptoms of a chronic dull pain are more difficult to evaluate and treat. This pain may never totally go away, but it can usually be relieved to the point where it is tolerable.

The first and simplest way to determine whether a resident is in pain is to ask. First, touch the resident and get his or her attention, then make eye contact and ask, "Are you in pain?" or "Does anything hurt?" or "Can you show me where it hurts?" If the resident with advanced dementia is not able to understand the meaning of the word *pain* or communicate the location of the pain, then a pain assessment tool is helpful.

Pain Assessment in Advanced Dementia (PAINAD) is a useful tool for assessing pain in nursing home residents with advanced dementia (see Appendix F). Developed by a team in a dementia unit of the U.S. Veterans Administration Hospital, it is adapted from an assessment tool for measuring postoperative pain in young children and from a research tool for measuring discomfort. PAINAD is easy to use, objective, reliable, and valid (Warden, Hurley, & Volicer, 2003).

All unresolved pain is reported to the attending physician; if the resident receives the Medicare hospice benefit, hospice nurses are notified. Hospice nurses are specially trained in treating pain and controlling symptoms for people who have terminal illnesses. If the attending physician or hospice staff cannot alleviate the pain, the services of other professionals may be needed. When the pain originates from the mouth, a dentist may be called to see the resident. If pain is unresolved by routine treatments, other physicians who specialize in pain management may be called for a consultation. The nursing staff should be aggressive in their quest to make residents comfortable.

The resident may have pain from an undiagnosed disease such as cancer. Often, when the resident is in the advanced stage of dementia, testing for cancer is not pursued because of the resident's limited life expectancy. Surgery is usually not indicated unless it is the only means of keeping the resident comfortable.

## Treatment of Pain

When the pain has been assessed for location and intensity, a treatment plan is developed with the physician and documented in the resident's care plan. This usually involves prescribing medications. Pain medications should be given on a regular basis to prevent pain. It takes time for a medication to be effective, and the resident will continue to feel pain for some time after the medication is administered. Pain medication should be titrated to a dosage that controls pain without producing significant side effects. Breakthrough pain can be treated with a pro re nata (PRN, or "as needed") order. Giving medications on a regular basis is more beneficial than dispensing medications only on a PRN basis.

Residents with advanced dementia sometimes experience difficulties taking oral medication. They may have problems swallowing or spit out the medication, pocket pills in their cheeks, refuse to open their mouths, or chew pills that are not supposed to be chewed. As alternatives, medication may be crushed and given with food, offered in liquid form, inserted rectally, or injected intramuscularly or subcutaneously.

IV therapy is a last-resort method of delivering pain medication. In fact, many nursing facilities transfer residents with IV therapy from a dementia neighborhood to protect them from other well-intentioned residents who try to help by removing the IV. However, moving to a new neighborhood takes the resident away from the team members who know the resident.

If the resident is free of liver disease, using nonopioid analgesics may be the first treatment choice for mild or moderate chronic pain. Acetaminophen is usually the safest and easiest way to begin treating pain unless the pain is clearly acute. Like any other medication, analgesics have benefits and risks that must be evaluated by the attending physician and side effects that must be monitored by staff.

When acetaminophen fails to provide relief, the next type of medication that can be ordered is a nonsteroidal anti-inflammatory drug (NSAID) such as ibuprofen. NSAIDs have serious side effects, including gastrointestinal irritation and bleeding, so monitoring by all staff is crucial for residents who are taking these medications. Because residents with advanced dementia cannot complain of gastrointestinal discomfort, it is often better to initiate an opiate medication only if acetaminophen was not effective.

Opiate medications are available to treat pain symptoms that are severe and have not been resolved by nonopioid analgesics or NSAIDs. These drugs, including codeine, fentanyl, and morphine, offer immediate relief. Morphine has fewer side effects than other medications, is effective in relieving severe pain, and can be given in small doses. It can be easily given in liquid form. Morphine is a widely misunderstood drug that many physicians are reluctant to prescribe for residents in nursing homes; nurses are uneasy in administering it, and families fear that it will cause their loved one to become overly sedated or addicted to the drug. Some believe that morphine will hasten death. Although it is often given to the resident who is actively dying to ease breathing discomfort, morphine will not cause death when administered in prescribed doses. The most serious side effect is constipation, which can be easily resolved. The Namaste Care nursing staff needs to become knowledgeable about all aspects of medication types including over-the-counter drugs, usual doses, methods of dispensing, and the conditions under which they are used.

## Monitoring

Once the pain is controlled, regular monitoring, following federal and state guidelines, ensures that the resident is pain free at all times. Some nursing facilities emphasize the importance of monitoring and controlling pain and refer to pain control as the fifth vital sign. Dr. James Campbell, in his 1996 presidential address to the American Pain Society, stated

> Vital signs are taken seriously. If pain were assessed with the same zeal as other vital signs, it would have a much better chance of being treated properly. We need to train doctors and nurses to treat pain as a vital sign. Quality care means that pain is measured and treated. (Fernades, 2010)

All team members should constantly monitor pain and discomfort.

## ACTIVITIES OF DAILY LIVING

### Clothing

Comfort care includes the choice of clothing for residents with advanced dementia. The simplest garments are the best because they make dressing easy. There are companies that specialize in clothing that is easy to use, such as dresses and pants with Velcro fastening. Namaste Care honors the dignity of residents by making sure they are well dressed and groomed. In the advanced stage of dementia, however, comfort is of primary importance.

Some comfortable options for women include soft sports bras or undershirts instead of traditional bras, slacks with stretchy waistbands, and comfortable blouses and shirts that button or zip in the front. Avoid garments that need to be pulled over the head.

Shoes are not necessary for a resident who is no longer able to ambulate. One facility found it practical to order several dozen slipper socks that were soft and warm and could be easily laundered. With nonskid soles, they are comfortable and safe for residents who need stability for transferring from a lounge chair to a wheelchair or a bed.

Shorts may not be appropriate even in the summer because residents' metabolisms change as they age, and older adults tend to be cold. Instead, consider pants with elastic waistbands and sweatpants.

Families and team members, especially care partners and nursing staff, may need to be educated about the reasons for residents to wear comfortable clothing. For instance, some care partners might feel that wearing slippers instead of shoes is undignified. They take pride in dressing residents to look their best and need to understand that it is more important for the resident with advanced dementia to feel comfortable throughout the day. If families disagree with this approach to clothing, their wishes should be respected. Some families insist that shoes are important; others do not like sweatpants. They may also provide clothing requests; consider the story of Betty, who loved her hat and white gloves (see page 110) or a request by one resident's family to have their father, who was a retired physician, wear a lab coat. Families' requests should always be honored. As an aside, I have heard from many directors of nursing and charge nurses that when residents are in Namaste Care, their grooming improves. They believe that this occurs because when a resident is brought to the Namaste Care room, the Namaste Carer often remarks on how the resident looks. This encourages care partners to want their resident to look their best. Before the Namaste Care program, these residents were often "invisible" (Simard, 2007a).

## Grooming

Comfort approaches should be used in grooming. In addition to washing residents' faces, staff can gently shave faces and brush or comb hair. Safe and appropriate procedures for these activities are described in Chapter 5.

## Oral Care

Oral care is very important for residents, and making the procedure comfortable takes sensitivity and special patience from care partners. Residents are usually not able to brush their own teeth and are at risk for oral infections, dental caries, and tartar buildup. The care partner should place a soft toothbrush in a resident's hand in the brushing position to see whether the resident remembers how to brush. The care partner might pantomime brushing his or her teeth as a memory clue. A child's toothbrush may be easier to use than an adult's toothbrush. If a resident is resistive, dipping a mouth swab in something sweet might help induce him or her to submit to some cleaning.

Assessment of the mouth is very important. Care partners should notify nurses at once if providing oral care seems to induce pain. Dentists are called if necessary for control of tooth pain. Extracting an infected tooth may be the only way to relieve pain.

Dentures may not be comfortable, particularly for the resident who has lost a great deal of weight. Judge the benefits and comfort of dentures and discuss them with families. When residents do not want to wear dentures, they usually find a way to take them out or to communicate their discomfort. Although some families may feel their loved one does not look dignified without teeth, most families agree to discontinue their use if the dentures seem to cause discomfort. Document the decision to remove dentures in the resident's care plan, and be sure to adjust his or her diet accordingly.

## Dining and Snacks

Care partners make dining a pleasurable experience, even if the resident needs extensive cueing or can no longer feed himself or herself. Residents are encouraged to eat as independently as possible for as long as possible. When they can no longer use utensils, finger foods may help residents to continue feeding themselves for a longer period of time. Cueing with simple instructions, such as, "Mary, please put the spoon in your mouth," and a demonstration of the action can be helpful. Make sure the plate color is different from the food that is placed on it. Consultation with a dietitian may be helpful to identify the best food consistency for each resident.

As dementia progresses, staff must watch residents closely for signs that they are pocketing food, which can lead to choking. If this is the case, physicians usually order special diets containing foods that are easy to swallow. If possible, the staff can ask families what type of comfort food the residents preferred, such as toast, ginger ale, macaroni and cheese, and ice cream.

Helping residents eat is a challenge for many nursing facilities when the number of residents needing individual assistance outweighs the number of staff. The regulations in all states prohibit anyone from assisting in the dining room who has not been trained in feeding techniques. Some states mandate that only care partners and nurses can feed residents. Other states require a special training program for anyone feeding residents. Assisting with meals should be a priority for all staff members. Suggestions for how to add extra hands and create a conducive atmosphere at mealtimes include the following:

- Train administrative staff and department managers to assist with dining, if allowed under state regulations.

- Stagger working hours so that extra hands are available in the dining room during the morning and evening meals.

- Play soft music during meals.

- Make sure dining assistants are talking to the residents, not just among themselves.

- Provide beverages for staff members so that they feel a part of the dining experience.

- Use clothing protectors that do not look like bibs, such as large linen napkins tucked under the chin, bib aprons, or barbecue aprons.

- Discontinue using institutional-looking meal trays.

- If possible, divide residents into small groups to cut down on the noise and confusion of eating in a large room. This can be done inexpensively with large planters or portable privacy screens.

To improve the experience of dining for residents with advanced dementia, a meeting should be scheduled between team members and the dietitian to brainstorm ways to make the experience of dining a more normal and comforting experience.

## Ambulation

Most residents in the advanced stage of dementia are not able to walk, even with assistance. If possible, residents should be evaluated by a physical therapist to ensure that there are no underlying physical reasons for the loss of ambulation. The staff should be trained in the correct approaches to maximize the resident's participation in ambulation or transferring.

When residents in the advanced stage of dementia are not able to safely ambulate, they are confined to a wheelchair. A regular wheelchair may be extremely uncomfortable for residents at this stage of life. The chairs are unbending and do not support the person who cannot sit upright. Each resident in Namaste Care should be assessed to make sure the most comfortable chair is available. Wheelchairs or lounge chairs on wheels that can be adjusted are the best choices. Geri-chairs with trays must be assessed to make sure that they do not function as a restraint. Residents enrolled in the Medicare hospice program can receive special chairs as part of the durable medical equipment benefit. Residents who constantly sit in one place are at great risk of skin breakdown, so Namaste Carers must be sure to reposition residents at least every 2 hours. Use pillows (consider special lavender-scented pillows) or rolled-up blankets and towels to position residents in their chairs. Asking a physical therapist to assess residents at least once month is a good idea.

## Bathing

Of all personal care procedures, bathing produces the most anxiety in residents with dementia. For them, bathing may be frightening and bewildering. Moving their limbs in the shower or tub bath can also be painful for residents with joint pain or contractures.

The first step in understanding how to make bathing pleasurable is to find out something about each resident's bathing history. Do they like tub baths, or have they always taken showers? Are they more comfortable and relaxed in the morning, afternoon, or evening? In many instances, the resident has been in the facility for some period of time, so the staff knows the resident's preference for bathing. If the resident is new to the facility, families can provide this information. Whoever is making the shower and bath list must understand the resident's preferences and then schedule the appropriate shift for that responsibility. Care partners must also be flexible. If a resident is resistive, staff may approach the resident at a later time or leave bathing for the next shift.

If possible, care partners should take the resident to the bathing area clothed or wearing a bathrobe. If the bathtub is an older model with a lift, hold the resident's hand while he or she is hoisted into the tub. Bathtubs that gradually fill and are easy to enter are the best option. Care partners should have enough towels available to keep the resident covered; if necessary, float a towel on the water to cover the resident or have the person wear a hospital gown.

Following facility bathing procedures, care partners should talk to residents throughout the bathing sequence. In a soothing voice, they should tell the resident what they are doing, ask the resident to hold the soap (if he or she will not eat it) or the washcloth, and make the resident feel that he or she is participating. Another approach is to talk about everything but the bath to distract the resident from the bathing experience.

Large shower heads, designed to create the feeling of being in a gentle rain, can make showers less traumatic. Handheld shower heads are also good to use, because they give the resident some control over the direction of the spray. Playing music during the bath or shower and making sure the room is warm help reduce anxiety and increase the comfort of bathing. Battery-powered radios are safer than plug-in electrical appliances in the bathing area. Also consider warming a blanket in a microwave oven to wrap around the resident after bathing. After the bath, staff should apply lotion to the resident's body and give a back rub. With a bit of ingenuity, bathing even the most resistive resident is possible.

## SAM

Sam was impossible to bathe. He did not recognize his wife of many years, and he did not want this "stranger" to assist him in the tub or shower. He was no more cooperative with home health aides. His wife was at her wits' end until she realized that her husband was a very sound sleeper, and she could wash about a third of his body before he woke up. Giving a complete bed bath took some time, but eventually he was completely washed! When he was admitted to a nursing facility, the care partners followed his wife's example and washed what they could before he woke up.

## Bed Baths

Bed baths are often the preferred bathing method for residents with advanced dementia who are resistive to tub baths or showers, are ill, have extreme joint pain, or are actively dying. Bed baths are comfortable and are given in the privacy of the resident's room. Bed bath techniques may need to be reviewed with nursing assistants.

To give a bed bath, first gather all necessary supplies; this includes soap, two basins of warm water (one for washing and one for rinsing), face cloths, towels, lotion, and dry shampoo. Clean clothing and personal grooming items such as moisturizer, combs, and brushes are also good to have available. Playing music and making sure the room is warm help to make the environment cozy and the experience soothing. Remember, bathing can be a pleasant experience; it just takes a bit of ingenuity.

## HOSPICE

When a resident progresses to the terminal stage of Alzheimer's disease or other irreversible dementia, it becomes evident that the person is approaching the end of life despite the best care provided by the team members. This final stage can last a few weeks, months, or several years. I remember one hospice nurse telling me that Mimi, a resident who weighed about 80 pounds and who barely ate or drank anything, would not die because she felt deeply loved by her family and the care team members. She was a "star" in the Namaste Care room, smiling at everyone with this twinkle in her eye that melted everyone's hearts. Her hospice workers visited three times a week to give her bed baths and take her for strolls around the facility. They called her "Mimi the miracle" because she would qualify for hospice, then begin eating again, and then have to be discharged from hospice. A few weeks later she was on again. One night when she was alone in her room, Mimi chose to die. Perhaps as the nurse believed, she could not leave when she was surrounded by so much love.

## HISTORY OF HOSPICE

The origins of hospice can be traced back to early Western Civilization when the term was used to describe a place of shelter and rest for weary travelers. Notations have been found among the writings of monks caring for warrior knights during the Crusades. They speak of caring for the aged and wounded knights, keeping their bed linens clean, serving warm soup, and washing the feet of the knights. Not much has changed; this comforting care is at the core of current hospice services.

The modern hospice movement began about 1967 at St. Joseph's Hospice in London's East End. It was in this hospice that Dame Cicely Saunders began to experiment with pain medication and symptom relief for terminally ill patients. In 1967, she opened St. Christopher's Hospice, a place of comfort for the terminally ill. This hospice became the model for hospice programs all over the world and mainly served individuals with cancer. I am privileged to have worked with the staff at St. Christopher's on a Namaste Care research grant. One of the nurses who knew Dame Cicely, as she was affectionately known, had a conversation with her just before she died. This nurse asked Dame Cicely if, looking over her life, she would do anything different. Her reply was that she would pay more attention to her patients with dementia. Dame Cicely died in 2005. Apparently even then Dame Cicely Sanders recognized that her patients with Alzheimer's had needs that were different from her patients with cancer and that this would be a growing population.

In the United States, Dr. Elisabeth Kübler-Ross began working with terminally ill patients in acute care settings. She found that physicians and other health care workers had difficulty talking about death to these patients. The patients, however, wanted to talk about what was happening to them and wanted to be assured they would be free of pain and would not die alone. In her discussions with dying patients, Kübler-Ross discovered that they usually go through stages in their acceptance of death. She reported her findings in *On Death and Dying*, published in 1969. This book, now considered a classic, heightened public awareness of the loneliness, isolation, and special needs of the dying. As awareness of the special needs of the dying increased, health care professionals and others turned to hospice as a way of caring for people with terminal illnesses.

A group from Yale University visited St. Christopher's Hospice in England and was inspired by what they heard and saw. They resolved to begin a hospice program in the United States. In 1974, a hospice home care program was developed in New Haven, Connecticut. An inpatient center, Connecticut Hospice, Inc., followed in 1980. This was the beginning of the hospice movement in the United States.

There are now thousands of hospice programs in the United States serving millions of people with terminal illnesses as well as their families. Some have retained their status as voluntary organizations; however, the majority of them are Medicare certified. Most hospice recipients have a diagnosis of cancer with a predictable life expectancy. Patients with dementia are a growing population of hospice patients and it continues to be a bit more difficult to make the prognosis of 6 months of survival, which is required by the Medicare hospice benefit. Lin Simon, Director of Quality at Gilchrist Hospice in Baltimore, Maryland, notes that "People with dementia get sicker inch by inch. They rarely have a dramatic change in their physical status, thus making a prognosis of 6 months difficult." (Spann, 2010)

A great deal has changed about hospice care in nursing homes and assisted living for residents with dementia since the first edition of this book. Today, I hear from nursing home care partners and nurses who are very happy to have hospice staff provide care as often as possible. With the acuity of care needed, extra hospice hands are welcomed! With emphasis on the physical, psychosocial, and financial burdens of hospitalizing people with advanced dementia, more physicians see that hospice can help reduce hospitalizations and readmissions.

I think some families still believe hospice is expensive and do not realize it is a program that their loved one paid for through taxes and it is their right to receive this benefit. It is still difficult for families, who have lived with the slow decline they have observed over many years, to come to the realization that the person they love is now in the terminal phase of Alzheimer's disease. Families whose loved ones have received hospice care are usually very grateful for the compassionate and caring attitude of the staff. They are also appreciative of the bereavement services offered following the death of their loved one.

The criteria for receiving the Medicare hospice benefit for people with advanced dementia is established by the Centers for Medicare & Medicaid Services (CMS) and change periodically (visit the CMS web site or search the Internet for updates).

One national hospice organization I have worked with, Seasons Hospice, has embraced Namaste Care and offers it as part of a special program for their patients with advanced dementia.

## NAMASTE HOSPICE CARE

Although originally created for long-term care settings, Namaste Care has been successfully adapted for use in nursing facilities and assisted living communities and as part of services offered to hospice patients. The following is an example of a hospice program that incorporated Namaste Care into its nationwide service program.

Russell Hilliard, executive director of Seasons Hospice at their site in Chicago, Illinois (and subsequently national director of supportive care for Seasons Hospice), contacted me in 2007 to ask for help in developing a program like Namaste Care for his hospice patients with advanced dementia. He had heard me present on the topic at a conference and thought that his staff, especially the nursing assistants, struggled with providing care to their patients with dementia who were sometimes resistive, had limited communication skills, and, if they could talk, lived in another place and time within their minds. He believed that the prevalence of patients with advanced dementia would increase, and he wanted to ensure that the best possible care was provided for them. This is how we adapted Namaste Care to create a special program for hospice patients with advanced dementia who reside in nursing facilities, in assisted living communities, at home, or in a hospice unit.

## Touch for All Seasons

Seasons Hospice wanted a unique name for their Namaste Care program. They invited staff to participate in the naming by submitting suggestions and then choosing the one that best suited their new sensory-based program. The winner was "A Touch for All Seasons," commonly referred to by staff and for the rest of this chapter simply as "Touch." Other hospice organizations using Namaste Care have retained the *Namaste Care* name, and I ask only that an organization that refers to my program by name maintain the integrity of Namaste Care. This means that it is more than just a marketing program to increase census and that it has structure and protocols as well as some way to monitor the quality of the program.

## The Touch Champion

Seasons Hospice recognized that maintaining the integrity of the program required having someone to assume responsibility for supplies and monitor the program. Therefore, every site or office has a "Touch" champion. Sometimes it is the supervisor of the nursing assistants, in other sites it is a social worker or music therapist. The champion's professional discipline is less important than his or her interest in the program; the main requirement is having the heart to help it flourish.

## Education

Education is the key to the success of any new program. Before "Touch" was implemented, a special education program was developed for the hospice interdisciplinary team and volunteers. Educating staff is expensive, and it must be time well spent. The "Touch" education was developed using feedback from many different disciplines.

The majority of nursing assistants and nurses in hospice organizations have some long-term care experience, and most have had some dementia education. Nevertheless, a review for all staff and volunteers of the fundamentals of Alzheimer's disease is valuable alongside instruction in appropriate methods for providing personal care using a "Touch" approach. Volunteers are not allowed to provide personal care, so their educational needs are different, as are those of social workers, marketing staff, and clergy. Seasons Hospice also employs board-certified music therapists at all their sites, and they provided a variety of ideas to enhance "Touch" visits using each patient's personal preference for music.

*Education on Alzheimer's Disease for All Staff and Volunteers*

The following topics were covered by the educational program on Alzheimer's disease and other dementias:

- History
- Normal memory loss associated with aging
- Signs of abnormal memory loss
- Early, moderate, and advanced Alzheimer's disease
- Medical issues
- Behavioral symptoms and approaches to use with each one
- Meaningful activities
- Assessing pain and discomfort
- Hospice criteria for patients with advanced dementia
- The "Touch for All Seasons" program
- Identifying patients
- Assessments (sensory and meaningful activity preferences)
- Creating the environment
- Long-term care facilities
- Home care
- Inpatient units (IPUs)
- Person-centered approach to care
- ADLs as meaningful activities
- Seasonal activities
- Religious issues
- After-death ritual
- Family support and unique issues experienced by families of patients with advanced dementia

*Additional Educational Programs for Nursing Staff*

- Assessing pain and discomfort in patients with advanced dementia using the PAINAD (see Appendix F)
- Providing personal care to patients in all stages of a dementing illness
- Medications used for patients with advanced dementia
- Identifying signs to determine when a patient is actively dying

"Touch" education is offered as part of all staff and volunteer orientation. A review of the "Touch" program is also offered once a year to all hospice staff and volunteers as an opportunity to review the program and share stories of their successes.

## "Touch" Criteria

The first "Touch" patients were those with advanced dementia, but as the program matured staff learned that it was helpful to any patient who could benefit from this special sensory approach to care. Patients are identified as appropriate for "Touch" by the assigned admission nurse or case manager and by the notation of "Touch" on the patient's initial care plan. A review of each patient's "Touch" care plan takes place at the interdisciplinary group meeting. At this meeting, any staff person or volunteer can suggest that a resident be considered for the "Touch" program.

Most of the patients participating in "Touch" have a diagnosis of advanced dementia; however, some other diagnoses have proven appropriate for the program:

- Late-stage Parkinson's disease
- Emphysema
- Agitated residents
- Depressed residents with other diseases or conditions
- Failure to thrive
- Debility
- Multiple sclerosis
- Amyotrophic lateral sclerosis

"Touch" Supplies

Each hospice aide is given a large bag with "A Touch for All Seasons" stenciled on it. The bag is made of material that can be easily cleaned. Aides take the bag with them whenever they are using the "Touch" approach to care. The "Touch" bag contains the following supplies:

- Gloves

- Ponds cold cream (a scent from the past)

- Q-tips or plastic spoons for taking small amounts of the cold cream out of the jar (these are disposable to eliminate infection control problems)

- Combs or soft brushes

- Noninstitutional tissue (which is softer)

- Hand sanitizer

- Lavender linen spray

- Hand lotion

- Small medication cups for the lotion to avoid cross-contamination

- Safety razors, shaving cream, and Old Spice aftershave lotion (scent from the past)

- Emery boards

- Fingernail clippers

- Seasonal items and aromas (lilacs and daffodils in the spring, roses in the summer, fall gourds, pumpkins, and the scent of cinnamon in the winter)

- A three-ring notebook with religious and spiritual prayers or sayings

- Fun objects, such as bubble used at children's birthday parties, puppets, etc.

- Small CD player and music CDs for volunteers and some non-nursing staff (Seasons staff have music apps on their cell phones.)

- Lollipops

- Pictures of items from the past to help initiate conversation

In an inpatient unit (IPU), supplies are kept in a home-like piece of furniture, a rolling cart that can be wheeled to patients' rooms. Most Seasons IPUs are units within a hospital, and they all have televisions that have a channel with soft music and beautiful pictures. Although this feature has replaced the need for a CD player in every room, there is always one in the cart along with a variety of music. Staff may offer supplies for families to use from the "Touch" cart. In one instance, a woman was actively dying, and her daughter was trying to keep her mother's mouth moistened with a sponge swab. When the daughter mentioned how much her mother liked sweets, she was given a lollipop from the cart and instructed to soak it in water and moisten her mother's lips with the lollipop rather than the swab. After her mother died, the daughter described the wonderful memories of her mother's last moments when she was sucking on the lollipop with a bit of a smile. Although the daughter had felt helpless to stop this terrible disease from robbing her of her mother, she was able to do something to make the journey a bit easier for them both.

## "A Touch for All Seasons" Lifestyle Preference Appraisal

A special assessment form was created for the "Touch" program. This form asks questions about special scents that the patient likes, such as aftershave lotion, or scents that he or she does not like or is allergic to. A patient may also like a scent related to a hobby, such as wood chips or cooking spices. It asks what name the patient likes to be called and about favorite foods and beverages. The assessment also includes the patient's likes and dislikes regarding personal care. For example, one woman loves to have her scalp massaged, another does not like her hair touched at all. The hospice aide completes the assessment after speaking with the family; if the patient is in a long-term care facility, the team members familiar with the patients are asked to help with completing the assessment.

## Creating the "Touch" Environment

It is not "Touch" unless the environment supports the program. The following are some examples of how "Touch" is used in different settings in which Seasons Hospice provides services.

*Nursing or Assisted Living Community*

Seasons staff or volunteers always knock on the door before entering a patient's room. They are trained to hesitate (stop, look, and listen) before walking into the room so that they may assess what changes must be made in order to provide an environment suitable for implementing "Touch." Are the lights on? Is the television on? How many people are in the room? These are a few observations they may make before entering the room. "Touch" usually takes place in a quiet, peaceful environment, so stopping to assess the current atmosphere helps staff and volunteers plan what changes should be made to create a suitably peaceful setting. If the patient has a roommate, that person must be acknowledged, and the hospice person will explain that he or she is visiting the roommate's neighbor. If the lights need to be dimmed and the television turned off, the roommate must agree to this change.

Of course, every situation is a bit different, and person-centered care means that the person comes before the program or how anything is usually done. One hospice aide explains that her Hispanic patients prefer the room to be bright, and another says that every time she comes into her patients' rooms the drapes are closed, and she opens them to let natural light come into the room. Such decisions are left to the individual staff or volunteer who has received "Touch" education. They know the purpose of the program and can therefore decide for themselves what the most appropriate environment is for the patient.

The scent of lavender is usually sprayed on the privacy curtain or on some fabric in the room to provide a pleasant smell. It is rare that a person does not respond positively to this scent, but it is suggested that the first time lavender is used it is sprayed on a tissue and placed under the patient's nose to gauge his or her reaction. Other scents can be used, as is fitting for a person-centered approach to care. For instance, a person who loved the ocean may be comforted by a scent from the sea; in the midst of a cold winter, a patient who cooked may enjoy the scent of cinnamon.

Hospice aides usually provide personal care ADLs during their visits; however, they are offered using a "Touch" sensory-based approach. People with dementia often are frightened by showers, so many times a bed bath is offered by Seasons Hospice aides. Supplies for a bed bath are gathered before the aide enters the room so there is no need to leave the patient. A hair dryer can be used to warm the sheets and towels.

## MRS. SMITH

Mrs. Smith was an 88-year-old widow who was in the advanced stage of Alzheimer's disease. She lived in a special care unit of a nursing facility. Her family visited on the weekends but had difficulty knowing what to do during these visits because Mrs. Smith did not recognize them and rarely spoke. Seasons Hospice staff completed the Lifestyle Preference Assessment with the assistance of the family and the nursing home staff and developed a person-centered plan of care by specifically recognizing what was important to Mrs. Smith before her illness. They discovered that she enjoyed gardening and loved to dance. She took great pride in her appearance, having visited the beauty shop every week. Her plan of care was to provide her with a spa experience.

When her hospice aide went into the room, she introduced herself to Mrs. Smith and expressed to her that she was going to give Mrs. Smith a "spa treatment." The aide dimmed the lights and played soothing music. The bed linen and privacy curtain were sprayed with lavender scent. The nursing home staff indicated that Mrs. Smith resisted any attempt to shower her; it usually took two aides, and Mrs. Smith screamed throughout the shower. Now the shower was replaced with a soothing bed bath. Mrs. Smith's hair was brushed with loving strokes and fastened with a favorite hair clip. She was told that part of the spa day was a facial; a warm, wet facecloth was applied to her face, then Ponds cold cream was applied, her favorite face cream when she was a young woman. Mrs. Smith's hands were soaked in warm water so that her nails could be groomed. When the "spa treatment" was completed, Mrs. Smith was dressed and told she would be going to a dance. Favorite dance music suggested by the music therapist was played while the hospice aide took her arms and did range-of-motion exercises to the music. Mrs. Smith was almost nonverbal; during her spa treatments, however, the aide reported that she laughed and one day even said, "I love to dance."

Mrs. Smith's family was told how they could make their visits easier for themselves and more enjoyable for her by brushing her hair and massaging her arms with lotion. Mrs. Smith had no problems with swallowing, and her love of coffee ice cream was communicated to nursing home staff and family members. This person-centered approach to care offered by "A Touch for All Seasons" made visits the highlight of the week for her family members, who wanted to treasure the last days they would have with their mother. Hospice volunteers are not allowed to feed patients, but they could brush her hair and massage her arms and hands with lotion; they also brought flowers and plants for her to look at and touch. Not only did Mrs. Smith's agitation decrease when the nursing home care partners replaced showers with bed baths, but she also needed less psychotropic medication. "Touch" created a better quality of life at the end of life for Mrs. Smith.

*Home Care Patients*

When providing "Touch" in the patient's home, hospice staff and volunteers try to create a soothing environment. The environment is made as peaceful as possible, just as in the descriptions of the nursing facility, and the same supplies are used. The patient may have his or her own CD player, or the hospice service may have given one to the patient to use even when hospice staff is not present. One day while I was visiting a patient with advanced dementia, an interesting situation developed.

## JAMES AND HIS WIFE

James was an 81-year-old man with advanced dementia who needed total care and was bedridden. His wife, who was also in her early 80s, was his primary care partner. This woman had suffered a heart attack the previous year, her sister had recently died, and on the day we were there she was caring for her 4-year-old great granddaughter. We realized that the wife needed "Touch" more than her husband! As soon as we entered the house, the hospice aide looked at her husband, who seemed fine and was sleeping. The granddaughter was given a treat, and the hospice aide turned on a children's program on the television in another room. Now it was time to care for the carer. We urged her to sit down in a comfortable lounge chair. The hospice aide took off the woman's shoes and tucked a quilt around her. We put on some soft music, sprayed lavender scent around the room, lowered the lights, and gave her a hand massage. The smile on this woman's face and her "Oh my" comment showed us that indeed she needed some replenishment. After the hospice aide finished massaging her hands and face, we encouraged her to rest while we cared for her husband. It was interesting that her husband showed little reaction to "Touch"; he was nonverbal and not very responsive, but his wife glowed and was truly touched.

As the "Touch" program grew, Seasons Hospice often found that the person-centered, sensory-based program was appropriate for patients who did not have a dementing illness.

*SAM*

Sam was a home care patient with cancer. The hospice aide reported that his home was always full of family members and that cable news was broadcasting on the television throughout her time with him. His attitude was usually, "Let's get this bath over with," and he rarely spoke as she provided personal care. The aide had just attended a "Touch" educational program and decided to try the techniques on this patient. She asked the family whether she could have some time alone with the patient, suggesting that maybe they could take some time for themselves and go for a walk. They seemed to be relieved and left the house eagerly. She then asked the patient what type of music he liked, and, much to her surprise, he said classical. After asking permission to turn off the television, she found some Bocelli arias to play on her handheld computer, and then she sprayed the room with the scent of pine, rather than lavender, because he had indicated that he loved hiking in the forest. Then she asked him to tell her a favorite story about when he was younger while she was giving him a bed bath.

She saw him relax as he talked about his life on the farm and how he thought that he was his mother's favorite. As she was bathing him, she felt that for the first time he seemed to enjoy himself. She then changed the bed linens, sprinkled baby powder inside his pillow, and offered him a drink. When she was finished, he gave her a huge smile and told her that he felt as if he was in a five-star hotel. When his wife returned, he said, "I'm as clean as the day you married me, and I feel cured."

The hospice aide communicated to the volunteers that Sam spent his childhood on a farm and loved growing things. When they came to visit afterward, they brought flowers gathered from their own gardens and fresh fruits and vegetables. This helped them find topics that he enjoyed, and the volunteers felt that their visits were—pardon the pun—more fruitful.

*Inpatient Unit*

The "Touch" program in an IPU is effective for patients who have a variety of diseases and situations. As previously mentioned, a cart was used to transport supplies for "Touch." In addition to the items listed earlier for the "Touch" bag, Seasons Hospice uses the cart to carry supplies for patients who are actively dying. The cart includes a Bible and other religious items such as a cross, rosary, yarmulke, and Star of David (see page 115). The cart also has information about typical signs at the end of life, along with suggestions for relieving these symptoms of impending death.

## DANIEL

Daniel was a 68-year-old patient in the IPU who was admitted for pain associated with prostate cancer with metastases to his bones. When I met him, his pain was controlled, but he was agitated; his body moved almost constantly. He did not speak to me but did nod his head when I asked permission to turn off the television and visit with him. I began to create the "Touch" environment, lowering the lights, playing soft music, and spraying his bedding with the scent of lavender. He kept watching me with his eyes wide open but not saying anything. I began to talk to him with loving words, telling him he was a very special man and how loved he was. As I spoke, I gently stroked his head and face. Gradually his body began to lose the twitching movements, and after about 10 minutes he fell asleep. His nursing assistant told me Daniel slept peacefully for an hour, the most he had slept since admission.

In all settings—nursing facilities, assisted living communities, home, or the IPU—after-death care is part of "Touch." If hospice staff is present at the death, they accompany the body to the hearse. In the IPU, a quilt and flag are available, just as in the Namaste Care program. The body is accompanied as far as possible. Some hospitals require the body to be taken through the basement, so the staff, especially if the family is also walking the body, will stop at the door to the basement or morgue area.

In the Seasons IPU located in Baltimore, Maryland, I had the pleasure of meeting the medical director, Dr. Harold Bob, who often integrates conventional medicine, Reiki, music, and aromatherapy. He has trained as a master in both Western and Japanese Reiki. The first time I made rounds with Dr. Bob, I was amazed at how he used his hands to assess and comfort the patients. He is a perfect role model for "Touch." This IPU has since trained several staff members to offer Reiki to patients.

Dr. Bob also led the way in changing the language used on the daily patient report. The staff now use *transition* in place of *die*, *dying*, or *dead*. For example, the daily reports on patients changed from "will die on unit" to "will transition in our care." The new statement more accurately reflects the hospice way of caring for people at the end of their lives.

## MARKETING

The number of hospice organizations in the United States has grown dramatically, from about 300 in 1986 to 5,300 in 2011. All Medicare-certified hospices must provide the same services, which makes it a challenge for hospice organizations to find an edge, a special niche in a crowded marketplace. Seasons Hospice believes that their board-certified music therapists (not reimbursed by Medicare) and their "Touch for All Seasons" have set them apart from other hospice programs.

My work with them continues to grow as we add refinements to the "Touch" program, such as a bag filled with Jewish items and one with Christian items to help trigger spiritual responses from patients with advanced dementia. For Seasons Hospice the "Touch" program is not just a marketing ploy; it has substance and offers a special service to patients with advanced dementia. It has enriched the lives of patients with dementia and those who care for and about them, whether professionals, friends, or families. I sometimes think of my work with organizations such as Seasons Hospice as sowing seeds, and it is a delight to see what blooms. A chance meeting with Russell Hilliard added many new blooms in the Namaste Care garden.

## NONTRADITIONAL TREATMENTS

Many nontraditional, holistic approaches can enhance well-being and provide comfort at the end of life. Massage therapy can be used to treat pain and discomfort of muscles and joints, for example. The gentle, relaxing strokes may offer comfort to a resident. Reiki is also gaining acceptance from the medical profession. This technique of laying on hands is used to create life force energy to promote relaxation. Reiki is not a religion and has no harmful effects (International Center for Reiki Training, 2012). Reiki treatments are being used in hospitals to accelerate healing, relieve pain, lower anxiety, decrease sleep problems, and increase appetites.

Acupuncture is another way of providing relief from pain. This ancient treatment is now being accepted by traditional medicine. Although no research has been done on its use for residents with advanced dementia, it is used to alleviate pain in rehabilitation and acute care settings (Berman et al., 2004).

Aromatherapy and the use of essential oils—especially lavender, geranium, and marjoram—may have calming effects on anxious residents (Flanagan, 1995). However, these oils should not be used on any resident with allergies. Aromatherapy is a natural, noninvasive treatment system. It has been observed that the aroma of lavender in the Namaste Care room appears to create a calming environment and may be one of the reasons why pacing residents are drawn into the room to sit and rest. Aromatherapy diffusers are available in activity catalogs and many stores that sell essential oils.

Patricia A. Young, director of nursing for EPOCH Senior Healthcare of Weston, Massachusetts, is trying a new initiative in her facility. Patricia has experienced excellent Namaste Care programs in two facilities where she has been the director of nursing, so she knows the emphasis on using lavender. She has made lavender patches (mixed with olive oil) from 2×2-inch gauze pieces, which are taped to the upper body of some of her residents who are prone to falls. The results have been encouraging. She noted at the beginning of one month that there were 19 falls. Then use of the lavender patches was initiated, and the falls during that month declined by more than half. Only one resident of the nine who fell was using the lavender patches. Additionally, she noticed a general improvement in mood and behavior for these residents. One particular resident had been given several different medications for her behavior and delusions and was too sensitive to continue taking any of them; however, when the lavender patch was tried, she became a different person, much calmer. None of the residents experienced any skin irritation from the oil. The goal, if the fall rates continue to decline, will be to discontinue using alarms on these residents.

Music is another way to decrease anxiety and lessen pain. Playing soft, tranquil music and nature sounds in a resident's room may help lower anxiety and reduce discomfort. Team members are always exploring ways to help residents feel comfortable. As long as there are no safety concerns and approaches are documented in the care plan, staff should be encouraged to try medical as well as nonmedical holistic approaches to alleviate pain and discomfort.

## COMFORTING ENVIRONMENT

Little research has been done on whether and how the environment of nursing facility residents with advanced dementia provides comfort (Calkins, 2003). Namaste Care is built on honoring the person in every way possible, so providing an attractive and comforting environment is important. Chapters 4 and 5 provide many ideas on how to make the Namaste Care room and a Namaste Care neighborhood look warm and inviting.

The residents' rooms, where they spend many hours, should also be as comfortable as possible. Rooms should be personalized with pictures and other familiar items; be sure to place these items where residents can see them. One enterprising facility painted the ceilings in residents' rooms with clouds and birds. Another facility repainted each room as they had funds available. Another facility asked organizations and private benefactors to adopt a resident's room. Some of the donations were monetary, and some took the form of volunteers to paint the rooms (see page 62).

Namaste Care recognizes that in order to maintain quality of life for residents right to the end of life, eliminating pain and discomfort must be a top priority. A palliative approach to care includes both medical interventions, such as pain and symptom management, and the more psychosocial aspects of care. Psychosocial aspects include the way residents are bathed and assisted with ADLs, how they are dressed and seated in chairs, and how meaningful activities can improve their lives.

When residents are comfortable, the staff feels better too. When residents are comfortable, families feel better about visiting their loved ones and are less anxious when they leave them.

## MATTHEW'S STORY

Matthew's family chose to discontinue hospitalization and not to pursue tube feeding when he no longer wanted to eat. His wife, Celia, and the Namaste Carers could tempt Matthew with sweet stuff that produced looks of pleasure on his face. They recognized that the end was near and decided to keep him comfortable and avoid aggressive medical interventions. Celia and Matthew's family wanted him to die as he had lived, with dignity and surrounded by people he loved.

Matthew's comfort was very important to Celia. She visited several times a week and said it was so much easier to leave him when he was comfortable and in no apparent distress. His half of the room was decorated with pictures of their five children and numerous grandchildren. Celia also bought a quilt for his bed.

Showers had always been Matthew's preferred method of bathing, and staff usually had no trouble bathing him when they showed him Celia's picture and reminded him that he had a date with her. As Matthew became less and less verbal, his care partners learned to read his nonverbal communication and kept him comfortable. He never appeared to be in pain, but staff members constantly monitored him. Matthew was dressed in clothing that was comfortable and warm. His family was reassured that he was at ease in his surroundings, which comforted his wife and children as they faced the loss of their beloved husband and father. They knew that he was in the capable hands of the Namaste Care team members.

# CHAPTER 9

# *Dying and Death*

To live in the hearts we leave behind is not to die.

THOMAS CAMPBELL

I have been in the long-term care industry for almost 35 years and have made friends with many residents who are no longer with us. So it was an interesting and very personal experience for me to write this chapter and revisit these friends. Many of their stories and my memories of them came spilling out of my heart as I wrote, and I thank them for the privilege of helping to make this chapter live.

When a resident begins to actively die, the Namaste Care™ program supports him or her in making the transition from life to death in a peaceful and dignified manner, free of pain and, whenever possible, in the presence of others. It is up to the living to help write the final chapter of the residents' lives. For the families, this leave taking will remain in their mind's eye forever, and the team members will do everything possible to make this memory as positive and serene as possible.

We often talk about a "good death," yet it is difficult to define because it is a matter of individual preferences. Most would agree that a good death is one that is pain free, yet even this is a personal choice. My father chose to have pain so he could still enjoy visiting with his friends who came to say good-bye as he was dying. Loretta Downs, founder of Chrysalis End-of-Life Inspirations, believes that a supported death is a good way to die. This chapter, then, is about providing a supported death for the resident, for his or her family and friends, and for the team members.

One of the ways in which Namaste Care can be expanded is to incorporate into end-of-life care the ideas of another program called No One Dies Alone (NODA), which is discussed in detail later in this chapter. The goal of NODA is to provide continuous companionship for a resident who is making the final journey of life alone, and it dovetails beautifully with Namaste Care.

Years ago, care of the sick and dying was the duty of families. Death took place at home with relatives, who were also the primary caregivers. Family members often prepared the body after death. People knew and understood that this was one of their responsibilities. Just as they assisted with the birthing of new babies, they also cared for the dying. Now, however, despite the wonderful work of hospice (see Chapter 8), many people with a terminal illness die in a hospital (Mitchell, Teno, Miller, & Mor, 2005), often alone.

In 2011, more than 5,300 hospice programs were operating in the United States, and an estimated 1.65 million patients received services from hospices (National Hospice and Palliative Care Organization, 2012). Despite the number of hospice programs and well-intentioned nursing staff, people die alone in too many cases. The United States is so large, and we are such a mobile society, that many times adult children live great distances from parents and are unable to be with them as they make this transition. Some residents do not have children; after one spouse dies, the remaining one is alone. In other cases, as people live longer, the centenarian may outlive family and friends.

Namaste Care encourages death to occur in the resident's home, the nursing facility or assisted living community. Transferring the resident who is actively dying to a hospital will not change the outcome. In fact, the trauma of moving the resident to a hospital may hasten the death. The nursing home is the resident's home, and the staff has become family—a family that is skilled at providing palliative care for a dying resident.

## MAKING THE DYING TRANSITION AS PEACEFUL AS POSSIBLE

One of the first signs that a resident is entering the last days of life may be a lack of response to activities that he or she previously enjoyed in the Namaste Care room. In addition, the resident will sleep most of the time and will be difficult to arouse. The person may not be able to open or focus his or her eyes when spoken to and may be uninterested in food and beverages; even the beloved lollipops are no longer tempting. At the approach of these signs, Namaste Carers shift their focus to providing end-of-life care for the dying resident and grief support for the family.

Dame Cicely Saunders, founder of the first modern hospice, remarked that "how people die remains in the memories of those who live on," and as part of the Namaste Care approach to end-of-life care, the room of the dying resident is made to look as home-like and comfortable as possible. During this time, it is beneficial for the resident to be in a quiet, comfortable place, away from the Namaste Care room. When residents live in a shared room, closing the privacy curtains will offer some seclusion. If possible and with their family's permission, it might be possible to move the roommate to an empty bed or some other room. This will provide privacy for the family and the dying resident.

Team members remove whatever medical equipment is no longer needed. They may place a colorful comforter or quilt on the bed and make the bed up with soft floral printed sheets for the women and plain colored ones for the men. Occasionally the resident who is dying has a slight fever, and a sheet is the only covering they can bear. Flowers on the night table and family pictures distributed around the room are also pleasant touches. EPOCH Senior Healthcare of Brewster, Massachusetts, showed me a room where a resident was in the final stage of life. He had been positioned on his side, and propped along the bed rail was a poster collage of family pictures and drawings that had been arranged by one of his granddaughters. She wanted to do something for her grandfather, and this was her final gift to him.

Appropriate religious symbols are placed in the room. A Catholic family might appreciate the rosary placed in the dying resident's hands, and Jewish songs may be comforting for someone of that faith. If a Namaste Cart is available (see page 115), it will contain music, a CD player, religious items, lotions, lavender spray, and other items that are useful for families and team members.

## THE REAGAN ROOM AND MILLIE'S ROOM

As discussed in chapter 4, nursing facilities that offer Namaste Care are encouraged to designate a private room that can be reserved for residents who are actively dying, such as the Reagan Room, named after President Reagan, who died of Alzheimer's disease.

Similar to the Reagan Room, EPOCH Senior Healthcare of Norton, Massachusetts, designated a private room that became available after the death of a beloved resident who had lived in that room for many years; her name was Millie. The administrator gave his approval to rename the room "Millie's Room," and whenever possible, actively dying residents and their families are offered this private and very peaceful room.

They also place a silk monarch butterfly on the door of any resident's room who is actively dying. This alerts staff that someone is dying in this room. The intent is not to discourage anyone from coming into the room; as a matter of fact, this alerts all staff that it is time to say their final good-byes, and they may just spend a moment asking the family whether they need anything.

## SIGNS OF IMPENDING DEATH

The Namaste Care commitment continues to honor the spirit within as the resident begins to actively die. The main focus is to maintain comfort, and all staff and family members are advised how to recognize signs of pain and discomfort (see PAINAD, Appendix F). It is important that those who remain, staff as well as family members, be honorable witnesses to this last miracle of life and take away positive memories of this death.

Nurses are usually the first to recognize when a resident is actively dying. They are often alerted by a care partner who has observed a significant decline in the resident's physical status or has an inner sense that the dying process has begun. When residents cross the threshold and begin to actively die, they may experience a significant decrease in their functional states. For example, they are

- unable to turn in bed without assistance
- incontinent of urine and unable to control bowel function
- difficult or impossible to arouse
- not hungry; eating or drinking very little or not at all
- unable to focus their eyes; eyes may have a glazed appearance.

It is hoped that all medical interventions have been stopped by this time. It is not appropriate for any diagnostic testing such as urine, blood tests, or X-rays to be given because they are uncomfortable and will not affect the outcome. Most medications should also be discontinued unless they are used for comfort. Oxygen may be used to help with breathing, but monitor for signs that the nasal cannula is uncomfortable.

In most cases, people with advanced dementia give signals when they are actively dying. Sally Smith (1998), a nurse practitioner working with residents in a nursing facility, has written about the dying process and identified what happens to the body in this last stage of life. She also provides ideas on how staff and families can care for nursing facility residents as they are dying. Team members should be aware of these signs and be able to show families how they can still provide loving care.

### Decreased Appetite

When the body begins shutting down, the need or desire for food diminishes significantly. It is believed that this is the body's way of protecting itself. Without food, there is no danger of choking or vomiting. When the resident stops eating, endorphins are released that reduce pain. Feeding tubes and hydration block the release of endorphins and can lead to discomfort. For several days or hours before the actual death, the resident often refuses all offers of food or beverage. Withdrawing from food and liquid is just part of the natural process of the body preparing for death.

During this time, the resident's lips and mouth might look parched. Care partners and the resident's family can help moisturize the mouth and lips area by using swabs that contain lemon glycerin or another moisturizing agent. Ice chips placed below the tongue or in the cheek and artificial saliva may also be used to provide moisture in the mouth.

A less medical approach might be to soften a lollipop in water and brush it on the resident's lips. A daughter told me that one of her last memories of her mother is seeing a small smile on her face as she tasted this sweet confection. Another daughter told me that she was using a swab with some type of lubricant when she looked at the clock and remembered that her mother always had a glass of sherry about this time. And so she gave her mother sherry once again, honoring what had been an important tradition in her life.

It appears that cold and sweet-tasting foods continue to be pleasurable, so small spoonfuls of soft ice cream may still be enjoyed by the resident and will help moisten the lips and tongue. However, it is important that care partners and family members watch the resident's facial expressions to determine whether any of these measures are uncomfortable for the resident. At this point, the goal is to provide comfort and pleasure. Food and liquid should not be forced. "Honoring the spirit within" includes respecting the right to refuse to eat or drink.

Some families have unresolved problems, and encouraging them to say "I'm sorry" or "I forgive you" might be helpful because this will be the last time they can verbalize whatever needs to be said while the resident is alive. A simple "thank you" and "good-bye" helps some families during this difficult transition. If family members are uncomfortable when they receive no reaction from their loved one, team members remind them that just sitting by the bedside is important. Families may also need to be reassured that it is all right to cry; it is an honest feeling and one that the dying person will understand.

Family and team members believe that they should be doing something and often feel helpless when the resident refuses offers of food. However, doing something is less important to the dying person than it is to the care partners and family members. Bill Thomas, a physician who began the Eden Alternative, expresses his feelings about what many perceive as doing nothing. He speaks of the difference between doing and being and how hard it is for most of us just to be. Those who are observing the dying process can simply be beside the person. They can be present with all their energy, and that is enough (W. Thomas, personal communication).

## Lethargy

As dementia progresses, the resident becomes more and more lethargic, sleeping for longer periods of time. When the resident reaches the actively dying stage, it will become difficult, if not impossible, to arouse him or her. This person will sleep most of the time. Namaste Carers and family members can read to the dying resident, play music the resident enjoyed in the past, and just be present. Staff and families are advised always to talk as if the dying person can hear them.

## Skin Changes

As the body begins to cease functioning, the heart rate may become rapid or may decrease significantly. The surface of the skin becomes cool and moist. Color begins to disappear until the skin appears almost transparent. The circulation of blood in the body is slowing, impairing the flow to hands and feet. The hands, nail beds, and feet begin to get cyanotic, turning bluish or looking mottled or blotchy. These are natural signs of impending death that can be frightening for the family. Tuck soft, warm blankets or sheets around the resident for comfort if he or she appears cold. I have used a hair dryer to warm the blankets, towels, gowns, and socks, but I do this in another room because the hair dryer is noisy. Soft socks on the resident's feet and warm lotion or baby oil rubbed gently onto the skin may also help the resident feel more comfortable.

## Fever

Occasionally, the actively dying resident will have a fever. This may be caused by dehydration or an infection. Fever can be controlled with medication if it appears that the resident is uncomfortable.

The resident needs to be observed closely to monitor pain and discomfort. It is difficult to administer medication when the person is actively dying; however, medication may be given rectally or in liquid form if the resident can still swallow. The best treatment may be applying a cool (not cold) face cloth on the person's face and limbs. If a fever is present, Namaste Carers should watch for it to break, because the bed linens should be changed at that time.

### Decreased Kidney Function

As the resident's body shuts down, the kidneys begin to cease normal functioning, and the body simply does not make very much urine. Urine output is smaller, and the color is darker. The resident has no bladder or bowel control, so he or she may be constantly leaking urine and feces. Even a small amount of urine or feces will make the skin tender, so it is necessary to check the skin frequently to make sure it is clean and lubricated. There is no need for a catheter at this point.

### Restlessness

Restlessness can be part of the dying process or an indication of pain or discomfort. Nursing staff should be asked to assess these symptoms and communicate the observations with the physician. Medication may be indicated to calm the restlessness.

### Breathing Changes

The respiratory system begins to shut down as the resident approaches the final hours of life. Breathing may become labored. Most people with Alzheimer's disease die of pneumonia. Although the process may not be painful for the resident, it is very painful for the family to watch. Morphine in low doses eases the breathing and will not hasten death. Oxygen administered by a nasal cannula can also ease breathing but may be uncomfortable, and it is important to monitor for signs of discomfort. Other medications can be administered if the resident seems anxious or distressed during the dying process.

Loose secretions in the chest are another symptom of impending death. This is not painful to the resident, but the rasping or rattling it adds to breathing can be upsetting for families to hear. Placing the resident on his or her side may help the fluid drain naturally. In fact, the natural dehydration that occurs is actually helpful in preventing fluid buildup. Avoid suctioning; it is uncomfortable, does not have any lasting benefit for the resident, and is not part of the Namaste Care approach. Remember that families will need constant reassurance that their loved one is not suffering, even though it appears as if the resident is experiencing discomfort. Sometimes playing soft music helps to mask these distressing sounds.

In the last few hours or minutes of life, breathing is very irregular and may even stop for short periods of time. This is called Cheyne–Stokes breathing and is normal at the end of life. Just waiting to see whether the person will resume breathing is an agonizing end to a difficult journey for the family. It may be helpful to the family to have someone else present at this time. Because family members may need to feel useful, encourage them to read from a Bible or other religious or spiritual book or to hold their loved one's hands. Team members should constantly reassure families of the importance of being physically close to their loved ones. Holding hands is a loving connection. Sometimes family members will want to lie next to their loved ones, a caring touch that easily communicates love when words fail.

When the signs of impending death appear, families may become frightened. They become alarmed when they see the changes in the body and do not understand that what they are observing is the natural process of death. Team members should help families understand the physical changes and assure them that dying is not painful.

## NAMASTE CARE PROTOCOL FOR ACTIVELY DYING RESIDENTS

When the Namaste Care nursing staff recognizes that a resident is actively dying, they may follow a protocol, such as the following:

- The nurse in charge of the neighborhood calls the physician to inform him or her of the patient's status and ask for comfort care orders. These may include orders not to hospitalize and not to resuscitate as well as orders for oxygen to assist breathing and morphine or other medications to ease discomfort. Ideally, these orders will already be in place and documented in the resident's medical record.

- The family is notified of the resident's declining condition by the charge nurse or social worker. If the facility has a private room available, like the Reagan Room, the family is asked whether they would like to move the resident to this room. They will be informed that if the resident recovers from this episode, he or she will be returned to the original room.

- A butterfly or some other symbol is placed on the door to identify that someone is actively dying in the room.

- When the resident is receiving hospice care, the hospice nurse is notified, and a plan to call the physician and the family is agreed on. The hospice staff and Namaste Care nursing staff must work as a team so that families are not confused by calls from the nursing facility and the hospice.

- With the family's permission, the dying resident's roommate may be advised of the situation. In some cases the roommate's family will be informed, especially if they visit often, so they will not be surprised when they come into the room.

- If a private room like the Regan Room is used, housekeeping is notified to make sure the room is readied for the resident's arrival. Before the resident is moved, soft music is played to welcome the resident, and personal pictures from the resident's room are brought into the room. Often, a plant or flowers can be borrowed from somewhere in the building.

- The medical equipment needed to make the resident more comfortable is brought into the room. Oxygen and personal supplies such as mouth swabs, face cloths, towels, and basins are stocked.

- If the resident is transferred to another room, the business office and nursing department must be notified. Regulations state that the resident's name must be posted outside his or her room. Bookkeeping records must also be kept current.

- The family is asked whether anyone else should be contacted, such as a close friend or clergy member.

- If a priest, minister, or rabbi is in the facility, he or she is notified that a resident is dying and is asked to stop by to offer consolation to family members. The family may want to have a special clergy member contacted, which would usually be handled by the facility social worker. If the resident is receiving hospice services, the hospice clergy person may be notified by the hospice nurse.

- The dietary department is notified so that soft ice cream, juices, ice chips, and other beverages can be made available for the resident. The dietary department also provides beverages and meals for the family and visitors.

- Social work staff members are notified so that they can make themselves available for family members of the dying resident.

Each facility providing Namaste Care should develop its own protocol; this is just a sample. A protocol is a valuable tool, especially when the charge nurse is new or not familiar with the procedures of the facility.

## Religious Beliefs, Traditions, and Culture

Before a resident reaches the last stage of life, the family should be asked about his or her religious and cultural beliefs and what they feel is important to the person. Religious and cultural choices are to be respected at this time. The Namaste Cart is stocked with a variety of religious and cultural items, including music, scriptures, and prayers for many faiths. When the nursing staff determines that a Jewish resident is dying, a rabbi should be called if the family has not done so because many Jewish communities provide bedside vigil sitters who understand the traditions of that religion for dying and after-death rituals. Catholics receive the Anointing of the Sick, formerly called Last Rites or Extreme Unction, when the nursing staff has determined that they may be actively dying. A priest should be called at this time. Because dying often occurs at night, when the social worker is not available, it is important to have this information available for the nursing staff.

## In the Presence of Others

David Kessler (1997) wrote about "walking people to the gate." Before September 11, 2001, travelers could be walked to the gate at the train station, bus station, or airport. They could wave good-bye and give a parting hug or kiss to their loved ones. Walking the dying person to the gate is a good way to visualize staying by the side of a dying person until he or she leaves. The team makes every effort to ensure that residents do not die alone.

Some families want to know when the end is near so that they can be with their loved ones; others cannot bear to see the person die. Some residents have outlived their family members, or families are not able to get to the facility before the resident dies. Many studies have revealed that older adults do not fear death but do not want to die alone or in pain (MetLife Foundation, 2011a). A study in Great Britain found that the greatest fear about dying was not the death itself but the idea of dying alone (Dignity in Dying, 2008). Most nursing facilities would like to provide someone to be with each dying resident, but without a structured program such as No One Dies Alone (NODA) it is a daunting task as care becomes heavier and staffing increases usually are not possible because of cutbacks in government funding.

## NO ONE DIES ALONE

Mother Teresa once said, "No one should die alone.... Each human should die with the sight of a loving face." Thanks to Sandra Clark, a registered nurse at Sacred Heart Medical Center in Eugene, Oregon, who founded NODA in 2001 (http://www.peace health.org), many people without families have someone to sit with them as they make this final transition. Sandra had the responsibility of caring for seven patients and one older man with a do not resuscitate order who was nearing the end of his life. He asked her to sit with him, as he was alone. She promised to stay at his bedside after she had checked on her other patients, but when she returned to his room he had died, alone. She resolved to do her best so that no one would ever have to die alone, at least not in her hospital.

Working with her hospital's volunteer group, she recruited a special group of "compassionate companions" to sit with patients who were dying and were alone. The program has spread throughout the United States and internationally. NODA is usually hospital based, but as soon as I read about this program I realized that it was desperately needed in nursing facilities too.

Those of us in long-term care, especially when we are part of a large corporation, are often frustrated by how long it takes to make changes. One of my roles as a consultant, and the one I love the best, is to implement new programs. In the real world this means developing budgets, sometimes finding space, deciding how to staff the program, and purchasing supplies; the to-do list before getting approval is seemingly endless. Then, I had the following experience at EPOCH Senior Healthcare in Norton, Massachusetts, which showed how quickly changes can be made. It beautifully illustrates how in just a few short weeks extraordinary changes can take place when you work with an extraordinary and dedicated team.

The story of NODA for Namaste Care began when a friend, Anne Sherman, shared a magazine article she had found that described a program called No One Dies Alone. Upon reading the article, I knew she had helped me find the missing piece for Namaste Care. It was a program that could make a profound impact on end-of-life care, especially for residents with no families. The article mentioned a guide for starting NODA, so I ordered it. The guide was written for hospitals, but I saw immediately that this program would be perfect in a long-term care setting, and I knew which community I wanted to try it with: EPOCH Senior Healthcare of Norton, which already had an excellent Namaste Care program and would like NODA. I was so confident that I requested a meeting with the administrator and some key staff to discuss it during a consulting visit just days later.

I met with administrator Kurt Wheaton, director of nursing Marie Bates, social worker Joan Woods, and Namaste supervisor and assistant director of nursing Karen Custodio. I gave a brief description of the program and how I thought it could be adapted for a nursing home setting. Their reaction was immediate: Yes, they wanted to be the first EPOCH community to pilot the program. The social worker remarked, "It's too bad we don't have the program in place now. One of our residents is dying, and she has no one with her." They looked at each other, and the administrator said, "I can come until midnight," and one by one they figured out how to be present for their own resident who was alone. They made it happen that night.

The next day, the administrator introduced the concept of the program to his department managers, and it was greeted with a positive response. They all agreed that, as a team, they could create NODA in a nursing home setting. New programs usually have a few people who question aspects of the program or feel they cannot assume additional responsibilities, but not this group. The director of maintenance, a man of few words, said, "This just makes sense. There is no one who wants to die alone."

It just happened that the administrator had scheduled his monthly general staff meetings for the next day, so he used it as an opportunity to introduce the NODA program to all staff on all shifts. At the end of the day I received the following message from him:

> Well, it's just past 11:00 PM and just finished my 5th and last staff meeting, discussing the No One Dies Alone program, and I cannot tell you in an email the full scale of overwhelmingly positive response this idea has gotten. Please call me the next chance you have to discuss it. In 3 of my 5 meetings staff members broke out in TEARS while discussing this. People here feel very strongly this is a program we need to do. You know that every time a program is introduced there is always resistance, but with this 100% of the meeting attendees agreed this is something we should do. When we talk, I'll tell you how things went last night with our actively dying patient. She ended up dying this morning at 8:20 AM, but we learned a lot about this program, just by doing what we could for her last night.
>
> Enough for now, excited to speak to you voice to voice about this. Thank you for bringing this program to us.

In a follow-up message that same day, the administrator for EPOCH of Norton explained how he would start to set up the orientation and sign-up process the next week. He said he had "strongly encouraged staff, especially my nonclinical staff, to sign up as volunteers. I told them that what I learned by doing this is that it is nearly impossible to sit with a dying person, at 1:00 AM, in a quiet room, a person that led a full, incredible life, and not come out a changed person." He also shared some of the reactions from staff when he had presented the concept of NODA to them:

> One team member's first thought was how great this would be for the team members, who often went home worrying about a resident who they knew was dying. She said she often called in after getting home to check on how the dying resident was doing, and said that instead she could text the sitter and get updates rather than calling and bothering the nurse. She thought *she* would rest easier at home knowing the resident was not alone.
>
> Staff commented on how much other residents would appreciate seeing us do this so they will know that when their time comes, we will be doing the same for them.

The story of Margaret tells what happened with the resident who was dying the day I first presented the NODA program to them:

## MARGARET

As Margaret was dying in her EPOCH home, her daughter was in Florida and son in Vermont. The very day that management was introduced to NODA, the administrator, Kurt Wheaton, volunteered to come in from 9:00 p.m. to 12:00 a.m. to sit with Margaret, and the Namaste supervisor, Karen Custodio, agreed to come at 3 a.m.

As it turned out, the son decided to come down from Vermont and arrived 15 minutes before Kurt arrived for his 9:00 p.m. shift. As the son was getting settled in, Kurt walked in, not knowing he was there. The son was blown away and exclaimed, "You mean you came in tonight just to sit with her?" He could not believe it. Kurt did not leave but stayed close by and checked on him every 45 minutes or so, brought a cold drink, etc. The son needed to get some sleep, knowing he would have a long day ahead of him, and he left about 11:30 p.m., extremely grateful that someone would still be there with his mother. Kurt remained until 12:30 a.m.

When Kurt left, he explained to the two nursing assistants and one nurse on staff about what was being done and asked their assistance in the 3-hour gap before Karen would arrive. The two nursing assistants decided that one would sit with Margaret as the other covered her duties. If the one team member who was left on the floor heard a call bell and could not answer it herself because she was taking care of someone, she would send a text message to the sitter, who would answer the bell and then return to her vigil. Margaret died the next morning, and she did not die alone, thanks to the team's efforts. It underscored for everyone how important this program could be to families.

The chief operating officer of EPOCH Senior Living, Joanna Cormac-Burt, had been copied on Kurt's messages to me, and she sent the following message to me in response to seeing them:

> This email has me crying! I have to say that even if we never get a minute of PR, this is the right thing to do and I am so overwhelmed with how Norton has embraced the program. Let's strategize how to get the program in all of our buildings. Kudos to you Kurt and your team! Your building embodies the EPOCH difference for which I am most proud and grateful!

With this endorsement, I heard my husband's words ringing in my ears from when he read Kurt's first message: "I guess that is your next program." I sat down at my computer, and a nursing home version of NODA began to take shape. With the help of Kurt and his team, the orientation program came together, and the first NODA orientation took place within the month. It shows how the right idea and the right team *can* make positive change happen very quickly.

### Staffing the NODA Program

As a hospital-based program, NODA is able to provide what it calls "compassionate companions," who are volunteers from within the hospital and from the local community. Most nursing facilities and assisted living communities, especially those that are for profit, have difficulty recruiting volunteers. Norton decided instead to recruit volunteers from its own staff, particularly because of the positive reaction Kurt received during the general staff meetings. As the program developed, volunteers could be recruited from other sources if needed. Brief meetings were scheduled with all staff to explain the role of a volunteer in the NODA program. The name chosen for these people was Companion Volunteers, and the following criteria were established for involvement in the program:

*Employees*

- Have been employed by EPOCH Senior Living for a minimum of 3 months and have the approval of their supervisor.
- Have a current tuberculosis test.
- Understand that they will not be paid for volunteering even though they are employed by EPOCH. If they are hourly employees, they will not clock in, and if they agree to stay after their shift, they will clock out before sitting with a resident or family.
- Understand that their primary role is to sit by the bedside of a resident who is actively dying, as determined by nursing, if no family members are present.
- May sit by the bedside even if family is present, if requested by the family.
- Sign up for times that are best suited to their work and personal life.
- Understand that they will always have the right to decline a request to sit with a resident.
- Agree to sign up for no less than 2 hours and no more than 4 hours.
- Attend an orientation and education meeting.

Several managers were enlisted to hold informational meetings with all staff. Forms were handed out asking staff to indicate whether they were interested in learning more, ready to sign a volunteer application, or not interested.

Each employee had to complete a form, including name and department, so that Kurt and his team could make sure all staff had attended a meeting. Meetings were scheduled for those interested in learning more about the program. Afterward, all those interested in participating in the program received a Companion Volunteer Agreement.

The first orientation and education program group consisted of staff who had decided this was for them and a few who just wanted more information before they made a decision.

### NODA Coordinators

Kurt and his management team decided that two team members were needed as coordinators of the program to ensure that at least one person would be available to take a call when someone was actively dying and could then call and assign volunteers. Assistant director of nursing Karen Custodio and social worker Joan Woods offered to do this. Each has a list of volunteers, their phone numbers, and the hours they could be with the resident.

### NODA Supply Bag

Supplies for a NODA program must be available to whoever needs them. Each program should designate a safe and easily accessible spot to store the supplies. For example, in the EPOCH program a supply bag is available at all hours in the social work office. All supervisors know where the bag is and have access to the office. The bag contains some of the same items used in Namaste Care, such as soothing CDs, a CD player, lavender linen spray, and hand lotion. In addition, they include religious or spiritual items such as a rosary, Bible, and poetry book. EPOCH Senior Healthcare of Norton is across the street from a Dunkin' Donuts, so a gift card was tucked in the bag for the volunteers. The bag also contains a "comfort journal" where volunteers can record their thoughts and note cards that can be sent to the family.

### NODA Orientation

The volunteer orientation begins with a discussion about a good death and what that means to each person. Most agree that not dying in pain and not dying alone comprise a good death. This is preceded by a general description of the program and some ideas of what volunteers would do as they sit by the bedside.

Each volunteer is given a Position Description that describes the process, from receiving the phone call and agreeing on a time to walking onto the nursing floor, introducing themselves to the charge nurse, and going to be with the resident. The Guide for Volunteers is reviewed, and each person is given a copy. Volunteers who are ready to make the commitment are given a confidentiality form to sign and a Companion Volunteer Agreement.

Orientation packets are provided for each volunteer, describing how to recognize that a resident is actively dying and how to tell when the resident has died. After the resident has died, volunteers are encouraged to sit with the resident if they feel the need to reflect on the experience, and then to inform nursing that they believe the resident has died.

Every person who completes the orientation at EPOCH is given a NODA pin; these can be ordered on the NODA Web site. Norton designed a certificate that they give to those who completes the NODA orientation, becoming official Companion Volunteers.

Volunteer orientation at EPOCH of Norton was scheduled several times during the first month because the interest was so high. It was offered during the day so that the majority of staff members did not have to come in when they were not working. This required the support of management to ensure that the volunteers' normal work duties were covered during orientation. I was surprised at how many staff members did come in when they were not working. I think this showed their commitment to ensuring that no resident would die alone.

## Nursing Staff

Special meetings must be held with the nursing staff to explain what is expected of the volunteers. It is important that nursing staff understand that even if the volunteer is an employee, he or she is not there to work. A team member who is volunteering is not expected to provide personal care to the resident. No volunteer is expected to do anything that he or she is uncomfortable with. Just sitting with the resident is fine; the object of NODA is simply to have someone with the person as he or she is dying.

Nursing staff at EPOCH decided that to activate NODA, the charge nurse and nursing supervisor will make a joint decision that the resident was actively dying. His or her attending physician is notified, and the family is called. If the family indicates that they cannot come in to be with the resident or the family requests that someone sit with them, the NODA program is activated. Each supervisor has the names of the coordinators, and their phone numbers are available at all nurses' stations. One coordinator is the lead, and if that person does not answer the call, the other coordinator is called. Each coordinator has a list of volunteers, contact numbers, and hours they are available to sit at the bedside.

The NODA supply bag is in the social work office, and all supervisors have a key for the office. It is given to the first volunteer and then passed to the others as they take their shifts. When no volunteer is available for a shift, the bag is left in the room, where staff can use it as they try to fill in so that the resident is not alone.

If the family is sitting with the resident, the nursing staff checks on them at least once an hour to see whether they need a break, food, and beverages or have questions. The NODA program is noted on the resident's progress notes.

Sustaining the integrity of any program is a challenge in any health care situation, because everyone is so busy. At EPOCH, they hold at least one NODA review in-service each year, and as the need arises for more volunteers, they hold volunteer orientation in-services. Information on the program is included in the orientation of all new employees, and after 3 months on the job, they can apply to be a volunteer.

The positive reaction from staff and families has made NODA part of the culture of this facility. When interviewed, NODA Volunteer Companions used the same words and phrases: "We are honored to be with them" or "It's just another way to show love for our residents." Whenever I visit the Norton facility, I feel honored to work with this remarkable group of people.

## COMPANION VOLUNTEER COMMENTS

Team member Felicia Jackson sometimes takes her 6-year-old son with her when she is volunteering. He knows that someone is very sick and going to live with God soon, and he seems to see dying as natural. One very special resident was dying, and even though the family was with her, Felicia wanted to be with this resident when she died. The family was very pleased that she would come in after her shift was over and loved having the little boy with her. They felt that the presence of a child was a reminder of the circle of life. The boy proudly walked beside his mother as they accompanied the resident to the hearse.

Dotti Raymond, business office assistant, told me that she has special things she likes to bring in when she volunteers, such as music she feels is peaceful and Bible devotional readings. She prays for the resident and talks to him or her about "going home." She makes a point of visiting even when family is present, and often they ask her to stay and help them with letting the person go, helping to make the transition. She is also authorized by the Catholic Church to give communion and is available to provide this sacrament for families as they sit with their loved one.

Denise Doyon has been a team member for 12 years and knows that sometimes the family can't be with their loved one simply because they can't bear to see them dying. When NODA was introduced to Norton's staff, she was one of the first to sign up. She feels that seeing her residents die peacefully completes the cycle of care for her. One of her favorite memories is of a resident who had no family present and was struggling despite the comfort measures provided by nursing. When her shift ended, Denise returned to the resident's room and held her hand and began to talk to her. Almost miraculously, she felt the resident become peaceful and slip away within a short time. Denise expressed a feeling that being with someone at the end of their life is an honor, something the staff at EPOCH of Norton just do naturally.

## SITTING WITH THE DYING RESIDENT

For nursing facilities that do not have a structured program such as NODA or hospice vigil sitters, here are a few suggestions that may help the staff provide someone to be with a resident who is dying alone.

- Ask department managers to take work, such as charting, to the bedside. At this point residents do not need conversation, just someone to sit with them and occasionally touch them.
- Notify the resident's church to ask whether they have volunteers who can spend time with the resident.
- Develop a relationship with a hospice program that will offer volunteers to be present for the dying, even if the resident is not a hospice patient.
- Provide special training to senior volunteers who are willing to sit with dying residents.
- Schedule a team member who is on light or limited duty to sit in the room.
- Ask all team members in the facility to sign up for 30-minute intervals.

The following example of a resident with no close family shows the commitment of the Namaste Care team:

*MAY*

> May had never married and had outlived most of her family and friends. She had one nephew who visited her occasionally but otherwise was alone. May had been on the Namaste Care wing for about 6 months when one of the care partners told me that she thought May was dying. When asked why she thought that, she shrugged and said it was just a sense she had that May was getting ready to leave us. A few weeks later, on my next visit to the facility, May was in the Reagan Room. Her pictures were hung on the wall, a rosary was in her hand, and a care partner was sitting with her.

Her nephew had been called, but he was unable to come, so the staff stepped in and became her family. One care partner came in on her day off just to be with May. It was moving to see this resident, who had almost no family and no friends, die peacefully holding the hand of someone who cared and wept as May died.

David Kessler (1997) stated, "Death by nature is one of the most isolating experiences we can ever have." Families who want someone to be with the dying person every moment may have unrealistic expectations. Team members should explain to families about the timing of death. From my experience and reading on the subject, when people choose to leave is a very personal decision. Families feel so much guilt when they leave the room even for a few minutes to go to the bathroom or get something to drink and the person dies. A friend's mother had a difficult time leaving her family, who were at her bedside constantly. One night this friend's daughter decided to stay all night with her grandmother and sent her mother home for a good night's sleep. The granddaughter told me that at some point during the night she desperately felt the need to go to the bathroom and then for no logical reason felt that she must brush her teeth. When she returned to the room, her grandmother had died. In another situation, a mother could not bear to leave with her children in the room. The following story is an example of this situation:

*JANE*

> Jane was dying of cancer. Her husband, Robert, their six children, and Robert's mother were in the hospital room watching over Jane after having been told she would not live through the day. It was a Catholic hospital, and when Mass was announced over the loudspeaker, Robert asked the kids to go and pray for their mother. As soon as they left the room, Jane took her last breath. She apparently could not die in the presence of her children.

My own parents taught me about choosing the time to die. My father evidently wanted me, his only child, to be with him at the end. Daddy was in a coma for many hours. Eventually, I needed to get some sleep and went home. As an only child, I had to make all the funeral arrangements. The hospital staff agreed to call me when he died. The next morning when I woke up, I realized the hospital had not called. I phoned the nurse's station and was told that he was still alive. I raced to the hospital, entered his hospital room, and lay next to him. I said, "Daddy, you waited," and he took his last breath. My mother, on the other hand, lingered until my father left the hospital before she died. I think she knew he did not want to see her die. Even with the knowledge we have about the last stages of life and the dying process, most experts agree that dying is as individual as each person's life experience.

If possible, someone should be with the family at the time of death, prepared for whatever emotions are expressed and ready to offer support. When my mother died, a nurse stayed with me, standing quietly behind me as I said my final good-bye. It was a good thing he did so because my mother's body began to move; thinking she was still alive, I panicked. The nurse gently touched my shoulder, explaining that this was a normal reaction of the body after death.

The team members must also monitor the reactions of family members as the dying process comes to an end. Tissues, some beverages, and a handy chair should be available for family members who look as if they might faint. Families, and even individual family members, differ in their comfort levels with the dying process. Some family members cannot touch the person as they are dying. In this case, the Namaste Care partner can hold the family member's hand and the dying resident's hand, connecting all in a circle of love. Others want to be as close as possible. The double bed in the Reagan Room is a wonderful asset to the family member who wants to lie next to his or her loved one. Team members are nonjudgmental about the actions and reactions of families during this time. Just as they are present for the person who is dying, they must also be present for that person's family.

## MATTHEW'S STORY

As a consultant, I am rarely with residents at the end of life, so it was an honor for me to be visiting on July 12 and to witness Matthew's death. When the Namaste Carer who had been staying with the couple was needed to help feed other residents, I stayed with Celia. We both held Matthew's hands and did our best to help him to the end of this voyage. Although not a nurse, I have been present at enough deaths to explain what was happening to his body. Celia became upset when Matthew's hands began to turn blue and his breathing became irregular. I suggested that she cover him with another blanket and hold his hand. Celia's face glowed as she held her husband's hand and told stories of their life together and of the special family they had raised. It was a beautiful sight, tears streaming down her face and love shining through her eyes. Matthew was a very fortunate man to have Celia beside him, literally "till death do us part."

Celia talked to Matthew as if he could hear her. She told him how much she loved him and how she cherished the years they had together. She told him she was fine and that, although she would miss him, she would be all right; he could leave with her love. Jennie, the charge nurse, walked in the room and realized that death was imminent, so she stayed at our side. Both Jennie and I were crying. How wonderful, I thought, that after seeing so many deaths we could still cry when a resident died.

Matthew would take a breath and then stop, and we would all think he had left us; then he would take another breath. This seemed to go on for a long time. Something seemed to be holding Matthew back. Then Celia told a comical story about their life together; we all laughed, and off he went on the wings of laughter. We hugged Celia, and she said her final good-bye to her dear husband, Matthew.

## WHEN DEATH ARRIVES

Death is always sad, perhaps heartbreaking, but a good death can be filled with reassuring memories of the last moments of life, with the gentleness and serenity with which a loved one slipped away in harmony with the world.

### Determining Whether the Resident Has Died

When death occurs, the resident will stop breathing; however, as the end approaches breathing may pause for a few minutes, then resume. At the end, breathing totally ceases. There is no need to immediately call the nurse because death has been expected and no medical intervention is called for. The resident's eyes may be open and the pupils enlarged; the eyes will not blink. They can be closed gently with a finger. There is no heartbeat, and the bowels and bladder may release. Each state has rules and regulations governing who can pronounce the death. A nurse should be called to determine the next steps.

### Families' Reactions to the Death

Some families want to stay in the room with the body for a while; others leave immediately. Making sure that the family's wishes are honored at this time is important. Death can be pronounced by either a nurse or a physician, depending on the state in which the facility is located. Families may need time to adjust to the death before a nurse or physician pronounces it. When family members are ready, they will be asked to leave the room while the body is prepared for the funeral home personnel. For the family and staff this is a time of conflicting feelings; sadness and a sense of relief are tangled together. Most families have lived with the disease for so many years that the finality of death, though painful, finally brings an end to the unrelenting assault of Alzheimer's disease.

Namaste Care is about care for the families as well as for the residents. Staff now is caring for the family, making sure the family members are not alone after they leave the facility. Many surviving spouses are elderly and may have health problems, so the staff should make sure they have someone to be with them before they leave the facility. The staff should evaluate the spouse's safety if he or she is driving home alone. At this time, having a friend or clergy member present helps put everyone at ease. When no one is available, someone from the facility should take the spouse home and stay until he or she is able to be left alone.

Families may be in shock after the death and not be able to remember things such as contacting their children, friends, or clergy. It is a very good idea for the social worker to make sure that all pertinent information is easily located in the resident's chart so that someone can assist the family in making these calls.

Some families are relieved after the death. They are exhausted from standing by as this cruel disease claimed the person they loved, bit by bit. How families react is very individual; team members should consider themselves to be shepherds guiding families along the end of the journey and ensuring their safety. Namaste Care continues after the resident has died.

## AFTER-DEATH CARE

### Autopsy

Some families decide to have an autopsy. *Autopsy* literally means "to see for yourself." It is a special surgical operation performed by a physician. It is done in a respectful manner in a laboratory or in a funeral home. Signs often posted in autopsy laboratories say, "This is the place where death rejoices to teach those who live."

The decision about having an autopsy must be made before death or directly immediately afterward, depending on state regulations. The reasons why people choose to have an autopsy are varied. Some families need to know whether their loved one really had Alzheimer's disease, a definitive diagnosis that can be reached only after the brain has been examined at autopsy. Diagnostic criteria are so advanced that brains studied after death show that 90% of the diagnoses of probable Alzheimer's disease are accurate. To be 100% accurate, an autopsy must take place. Results are available within 3 months.

Some residents are enrolled in research programs that have an autopsy as part of their protocol. In those cases, the facility should have the information about whom to inform when the resident has died so that the autopsy can be done within the appropriate time frame.

One of the greatest fears of families considering autopsy is that the body will be disfigured. This is not true. An incision is made in the back of the scalp, and the scar is not visible. Most religions allow this procedure. If the family is in doubt, their religious or spiritual adviser can assist in making the decision.

## Brain and Organ Donation

Donating a brain or any other part of the body to research may be some residents' final gift. If someone does choose to donate a part of his or her body to research, the team members should be informed by the family to ensure that the person's wishes are carried out. The Alzheimer's Association has information about brain autopsy, and many research centers also have literature about donations. The medical record should contain information about the resident's wish to make an organ donation and instructions on disposition of the body.

## Preparing the Body

The Namaste Care nursing staff prepares the body for the funeral home, following the facility's nursing procedures. If the family was not with the resident when he or she died, the nurse needs to call and inform them about the death. Family members are asked whether they want to see the body before the funeral home is called. Sometimes, they are on their way to the facility when the resident dies. In these cases, the team members prepare the room and the resident so that everything looks as peaceful as possible.

The resident is cleaned and dressed in fresh pajamas or a night-gown, not a hospital gown. Hair is combed and neatly groomed. After a person dies, the skin takes on a grayish hue; the face is devoid of color. A bit of light lipstick for women and a touch of rouge can improve the appearance of the skin. All medical equipment is taken from the room. Music is playing, and lights are dimmed. An over-the-bed table containing the resident's personal pictures and flowers is a nice touch.

When the family arrives, someone from the Namaste Care team who feels particularly close to the family, or the person who was with the resident as he or she died, walks into the room with the family. Tissues should be available. Family members are asked whether they want someone to stay in the room with them or whether they want to be alone. Some families need someone to be with them. Others just need to be alone. If families want to be left alone, have a team member check in periodically.

## Taking the Resident Out of the Facility

Years ago, residents' bodies were hidden from other residents as the gurney was being wheeled out of the facility. When a death occurred, residents were taken to their rooms, and all the doors were shut. The body would be quickly wheeled through the corridor, and then staff would let everyone out of their rooms. Of course, the first question out of the residents' mouths was, "Who died?"

The subject of death, though not completely out of the shadows, is taking steps toward the light of reality. Death is not a fearful subject for the residents, and honoring residents' bodies as they leave the facility is not upsetting for residents. The Namaste Care ritual honors residents even after death has occurred and they are leaving the facility.

When the body is ready to leave the room, team members place a quilt or flag over it. Supervisors know where "the box" is located. In the box are a quilt and a flag. Some Namaste Care facilities have a quilt made just for this purpose, with strips of a light fabric that staff can sign with a laundry marker. Others just purchase a beautiful quilt and have all staff members sign it. In larger facilities, each floor has "the box," and the quilt is signed by staff on that floor or neighborhood. The flag is draped over the body if the resident was a veteran. A note in the resident's medical record, usually found in the social history, should contain the person's military information.

The gurney is wheeled out, accompanied by family, friends, and staff. Sometimes a prayer is read or a song is offered as the gurney is being placed in the hearse. Most of the time, the team member walking beside the gurney places his or her hand on the body, reassuring the resident that even in death he or she is not alone. The quilt or flag is taken off the gurney as it is being placed in the hearse and returned to "the box" because it does not touch the body and therefore does not need to be washed.

Rabbi Carol of Life Choice Hospice in Massachusetts wrote this poem for team members to use as they place the quilt over the body.

## A Final Blessing

As flowers cover the earth outside
As leaves fall from the tree in autumn
We cover you with this quilt of colors
May it keep you warm
May it be your guide
Shalom, my friend
Day is done
May you rest in peace.
Amen

## MATTHEW'S STORY

> After Matthew died, Celia requested some time alone with her husband. When she was ready to leave the room, Namaste Care team members came in to clean and dress Matthew. All medical equipment was taken from the room, and the bedside table was arranged with his pictures, a live plant, and a small flag to pay homage to his years of service in the military. Celia then sat with him until the funeral home attendants arrived. She left the room while his body was put on the gurney. An American flag was placed over Matthew, and with his wife, Celia, the charge nurse, a care partner, and other team members, he left the place that had been his home for several years. As they walked alongside the gurney, everyone touched Matthew. When they reached the hearse, the gurney was placed in the back, and the Namaste Carer read a brief poem. Then, at this very sad moment when the hearse was leaving, everyone spontaneously waved; realizing what they had done, they laughed and cried and hugged each other as Matthew was slowly driven away.

Celia later remarked that the experience of her husband's death was beautiful, even peaceful. She was so surprised that although sad, she felt honored that staff was with her and shared the final moments. Accompanying Matthew to the hearse provided her with a sense of closure, and she had an overwhelming feeling of peace. She said, "I'm glad I stayed to the end. I would not have wanted to miss this last part of our journey together."

I found an interesting tradition in the United Kingdom: The hearse starts the last journey at the care home where friends and family have gathered, or the hearse drives by the care home so that staff can say good-bye to the resident. After the burial, the wake may also be held in the care home.

After the deceased resident is taken from the building, Namaste Care continues. The bed is stripped and remade with a bedspread and pillow. Namaste Care team members often talk about how sad they feel if the bed is left unmade after a resident they have cared for dies; there is nothing to show that a person lived and died in that room. Instead, care partners make the bed with just a bedspread (because fresh linen will be needed when a new resident is admitted) and place a silk rose on the bed along with a picture or some other personal item of the resident. Usually, management allows this memorial to stay on the bed for at least 24 hours. This seems to help the staff grieve; it gives everyone time to adjust to the death before another resident is moved to the bed.

Clothing and other personal items are packed in boxes, never garbage bags, and stored in a safe place until the family is available to pick them up or indicates that they should be donated to other residents.

## Taking Care of the Team Members

After the resident has left the building, someone needs to thank the team members for the loving care they have given to the resident. The charge nurse usually gathers the facility staff for this acknowledgment and also informs the incoming staff members of the death, thanking them for their care as well. It is helpful for the team members, many of whom feel as if they have lost a friend or relative, to hear the positive details about the death, such as that the resident died peacefully and was surrounded by family, staff, or volunteers. Even though they deal with death more than the average person, all team members still need reassurance that the death was a good death and that they made a difference in the quality of life and death of the resident.

We must never forget how much the staff cares about the residents. Many staff members need to talk about favorite residents long after a death has occurred. One resident who paced all day unless he was coaxed into the Namaste Care room is always remembered when the Namaste Carers look at "his" couch. His spirit remains in the thoughts of staff, as do the spirits of so many residents who have lived and died in nursing facilities.

## BEREAVEMENT SERVICES

Within a day after the death, the social worker should circulate a sympathy card on the neighborhood and ask all team members to sign it. Department managers and the administrator should also sign it. Make sure that someone from the facility can attend the funeral or the viewing; it is a gesture that means so much to the family and is helpful to the grieving staff.

## EVALUATING CARE

Several days after the death, a brief meeting must be held for each shift that helped care for the deceased resident. The purpose is to evaluate the effectiveness of the Namaste Care approach to the dying process. Facilitated by the social worker or charge nurse, the team members are asked questions about the resident's time in Namaste Care and whether the resident's death was

- Pain free
- Peaceful
- Without signs of distress
- With family, staff, and volunteers present and supported

We want to learn what we could have done better and what went well. It is very important that we always end with positive comments. At the end of the meeting, the resident is honored with a brief period of silence; then, memories of the resident are shared. These usually produce laughter, and the meeting ends, much as our friend Matthew's life did, with joy. It is my fervent wish that everyone living with dementia can experience the equivalent of Matthew's good death.

### MATTHEW'S STORY

After Matthew's death, the grieving process began with small reminders to staff that Matthew Wilk had lived and died in the Reagan Room. Namaste Care team members were thanked by the family and by department managers for their part in helping to make Matthew's death a good death. A memorial service was held later in the week.

# Epilogue

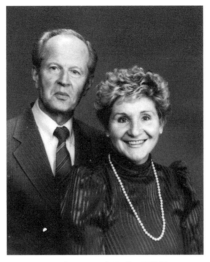

Matthew and Celia Wilk.

"Do not go where the path may lead, go instead
where there is no path and leave a trail."

Ralph Waldo Emerson

When I began doing Namaste Care™, I never imagined how far-reaching its impact would be and that it would touch so many lives. In writing the second edition of this book, I was also surprised to realize how many changes have occurred in the design and implementation of the Namaste Care program in the 7 years since the first edition published. For example, Namaste Care is now international and revisions to this edition reflect differences in implementing the program in other countries. Yet end-of-life care is truly a worldwide issue and Namaste Care, with its "loving touch" approach to care, transcends language and culture.

Namaste Care shows how you can make a difference in the lives of people with dementia . . . so leave a trail!

Namaste, Joyce

# Namaste Care Nursing Supplies

## PERSONAL SUPPLIES

Each resident who attends Namaste Care™ on a regular basis must have a zip-lock plastic bag clearly marked with his or her name. The bag should contain the following personal care items:

- Hairbrush and/or comb
- Nail clipper
- Emory board
- Lip balm
- Any other personal items supplied by the family (e.g., lipstick, additional make-up, hair decorations, after-shave lotion)

## GENERAL SUPPLIES

### Hair Products

- Combs and/or brushes
- Ribbons, decorative hair combs, other washable hair ornaments for the ladies

### Face Products

- Face cream, unscented and nonallergenic (Ponds is a favorite). For infection control, cream must be transferred into individual containers or scooped from the original container using individual Q-tips or other applicators before putting it on residents' faces
- Shaving cream (same infection precautions apply as for face cream)

- Safety razor (must have a safe and appropriate container for disposing of razors)
- Shaving lotion (Old Spice is a favorite). Ask the family about the resident's preferred brand of after-shave lotion (the family may provide it)

## Mouth Care Products

- Lemon glycerin swab sticks
- Toothette disposable oral swabs
- Lip gloss

## Hand and Fingernail Products

- Basins
- Soap
- Orange sticks
- Emory boards
- Nail clippers

## Skin Products

- Baby oil or lotions
- Unscented lotions

## Food and Beverages

- Thickeners
- Yogurt
- Ice cream
- Pudding
- Lollipops
- Orange slices
- Crushed pineapple
- Popsicles

- Orange juice
- Cranberry juice
- Soft cookies

## Paper Products
- Paper cups
- Covered sip cups
- Flexible straws
- Spoons
- Napkins
- Plastic wrap
- Markers and labels
- Small storage bags
- Paper towels

## Linen
- Pillows (for positioning)
- Blankets (colorful)
- Sheets (colorful)
- Quilts
- Face cloths
- Towels

## Miscellaneous
- Disposable wipes
- Small plastic bags for individual residents
- Large plastic bags for storing items
- Wastebasket and plastic inserts
- Laundry basket for soiled items
- Latex gloves

- Hand-washing liquid
- Pens and pencils
- Laundry marker
- Notepaper
- Communication book

# Namaste Care Activity Supplies

## ACTIVITY SUPPLIES

- Stuffed animals, especially soft, realistic birds that make specific bird calls
- Realistic dolls
- Aromatherapy diffuser (must be approved by maintenance department)
- Essential oils, especially lavender
- Scents that reflect different seasons, such as fir and cinnamon for winter, cut grass and flowers for spring/summer, and pumpkin for autumn
- Nature videos
- Sensory materials (e.g., pieces of fabric, silk, satin, leather, rabbit fur, lace, cashmere)
- Antique items (e.g., kitchen implements, marbles, old glass milk bottles, recipe boxes)
- Musical items (e.g., wind chimes, music boxes, rain sticks, drums, bells, singing bowl)
- Portable CD/tape player/digital media player
- Compact disks (CDs) or audiotapes of music and nature sounds
- Tabletop fountains
- Assorted reading material, including spiritual texts, poetry, holiday readings
- Humorous material (e.g., funny hats, circus wigs, realistic animal puppets)
- Sensory balls
- Bubble soap and a bubble machine

# Namaste Care Resources

## ALZHEIMER'S INFORMATION AND EDUCATION

Alzheimer's Association (United States headquarters). Information about local Alzheimer's Association chapters is available on the national headquarters web site.

http://www.alz.org

Alzheimer's Disease Education and Referral Center (ADEAR)

http://www.alzheimers.org

Alzheimer Europe

http://www.alzheimer-europe.org/EN

Alzheimer's Society

http://alzheimers.org.uk

Alzheimer Scotland

http://www.alzscot.org

Alzheimer's Association Australia

http://www.health.wa.gov.au/services/detail.cfm?Unit_ID=865

Alzheimer's Disease International

http://www.alz.co.uk

Dementia Care Matters

http://www.dementiacarematters.com

## SPECIAL RESOURCES

There are numerous web sites devoted to issues surrounding end-of-life care. In addition to the sites listed below, you can do an Internet search of any of the following key words:

- Hospice care
- Palliative care

- Death and dying
- Advanced dementia
- End-of-life care

| | |
|---|---|
| Good Endings | http://www.goodendings.net |
| National Hospice and Palliative Care Organization (NHPCO) | http://www.nhpco.org |

Local hospices are listed in your local yellow pages or on the Internet (search using the name of your city followed by *hospice* to find services in your area).

## ACTIVITY SUPPLIES

| | |
|---|---|
| Nasco | http://www.enasco.com |
| Best Alzheimer's Products | http://www.best-alzheimers-products.com |
| S&S Worldwide | http://www.ssww.com/therapy-and-rehab |
| Alternative Solutions in Long Term Care LLC | http://www.activitytherapy.com/dementiastore.htm |
| Cedar Lake Nature Series | http://www.cedarlakedvd.com |
| Elder Song Publications, Inc. | http://www.eldersong.com |

# Namaste Care Activities of Daily Living Checklist

| Resident Name: | | | | | | | | | | | | | | | |
|---|---|---|---|---|---|---|---|---|---|---|---|---|---|---|---|
| **Date** | 1 | 2 | 3 | 4 | 5 | 6 | 7 | 8 | 9 | 10 | 11 | 12 | 13 | 14 | 15 |
| Face washed and lotioned | | | | | | | | | | | | | | | |
| Hands washed and lotioned | | | | | | | | | | | | | | | |
| Feet washed and lotioned | | | | | | | | | | | | | | | |
| Fingernails cleaned and clipped | | | | | | | | | | | | | | | |
| Hair brushed | | | | | | | | | | | | | | | |
| Snack | | | | | | | | | | | | | | | |
| Beverage | | | | | | | | | | | | | | | |
| Range of motion | | | | | | | | | | | | | | | |
| Reading | | | | | | | | | | | | | | | |
| Seasonal scents | | | | | | | | | | | | | | | |
| Family friend visit | | | | | | | | | | | | | | | |
| Awake 50% of time | | | | | | | | | | | | | | | |
| Appears happy | | | | | | | | | | | | | | | |

**Resident Name:**

| Date | 16 | 17 | 18 | 19 | 20 | 21 | 22 | 23 | 24 | 25 | 26 | 27 | 28 | 29 | 30 | 31 |
|---|---|---|---|---|---|---|---|---|---|---|---|---|---|---|---|---|
| Face washed and lotioned | | | | | | | | | | | | | | | | |
| Hands washed and lotioned | | | | | | | | | | | | | | | | |
| Feet washed and lotioned | | | | | | | | | | | | | | | | |
| Fingernails cleaned and clipped | | | | | | | | | | | | | | | | |
| Hair brushed | | | | | | | | | | | | | | | | |
| Snack | | | | | | | | | | | | | | | | |
| Beverage | | | | | | | | | | | | | | | | |
| Range of motion | | | | | | | | | | | | | | | | |
| Reading | | | | | | | | | | | | | | | | |
| Seasonal scents | | | | | | | | | | | | | | | | |
| Family friend visit | | | | | | | | | | | | | | | | |
| Awake 50% of the time | | | | | | | | | | | | | | | | |
| Appears happy | | | | | | | | | | | | | | | | |

# DEMENTIA
# BILL *of*
# RIGHTS

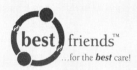

*Every person diagnosed with Alzheimer's disease or other dementia deserves:*

- To be informed of one's diagnosis
- To have appropriate, ongoing medical care
- To be treated as an adult, listened to, and afforded respect for one's feelings and point of view
- To be with individuals who know one's life story, including cultural and spiritual traditions
- To experience meaningful engagement throughout the day
- To live in a safe and stimulating environment
- To be outdoors on a regular basis
- To be free from psychotropic medications whenever possible
- To have welcomed physical contact, including hugging, caressing, and handholding
- To be an advocate for oneself and for others
- To be part of a local, global, or online community
- To have care partners well trained in dementia care

The Best Friends™ Dementia Bill of Rights by Virginia Bell & David Troxel. Copyright © 2013 Health Professions Press, Inc.

# Pain Assessment in Advanced Dementia (PAINAD) Scale

Name_____     Date_____

| | 0 | 1 | 2 | Score |
|---|---|---|---|---|
| **Breathing (independent of vocalization)** | Normal | Occasional labored breathing<br>Short period of hyperventilation | Noisy labored breathing<br>Long period of hyperventilation<br>Cheyne-Stokes respiration | |
| **Negative Vocalization** | None | Occasional moan or groan<br>Low-level speech with a negative or disapproving quality | Repeated, troubled calling out<br>Loud moaning or groaning<br>Crying | |
| **Facial Expression** | Smiling, or inexpressive | Sad<br>Frightened<br>Frowning | Facial grimacing | |
| **Body Language** | Relaxed | Tense<br>Distressed pacing<br>Fidgeting | Rigid<br>Clenched fists<br>Knees pulled up<br>Pulling or pushing away<br>Striking out | |
| **Consolability** | No need to console | Distracted or reassured by voice or touch | Unable to console, distract, or reassure | |
| | | | **TOTAL** | |

Signature_____

Source: Warden, V., Hurley, A.C., & Volicer, L. (2003). Development and psychometric evaluation of the PAINAD (Pain Assessment in Advanced Dementia) Scale. *Journal of the American Medical Directors Association, 4*, 9–15. Reprinted with permission.

## KEY

### Breathing

1. *Normal breathing* is characterized by effortless, quiet, rhythmic (smooth) respirations.

2. *Occasional labored breathing* is characterized by episodic bursts of harsh, difficult, or straining respirations.

3. *Short period of hyperventilation* is characterized by intervals of rapid, deep breaths lasting a short period of time.

4. *Noisy labored breathing* is characterized by negative sounding respirations on inhalation or exhalation. These may be loud, gurgling, or wheezing and appear strenuous or straining.

5. *Long period of hyperventilation* is characterized by an excessive rate and depth of respiration lasting a considerable time.

6. *Cheyne-Stokes respiration* is characterized by rhythmic waxing and waning of breathing, from very deep to shallow respirations with periods of apnea (cessation of breathing).

### Negative Vocalization

1. *None* is characterized by speech or vocalization that has a neutral or pleasant quality.

2. *Occasional moan or groan* is characterized by mournful or murmuring sounds, wails, or laments. Groaning is characterized by louder than usual, inarticulate involuntary sounds, often abruptly beginning and ending.

3. *Low-level speech with a negative or disapproving quality* is characterized by muttering, mumbling, whining, grumbling, or swearing in a low volume with a complaining, sarcastic, or caustic tone.

4. *Repeated, troubled calling out* is characterized by phrases or words being used over and over in a tone that suggests anxiety, uneasiness, or distress.

5. *Loud moaning or groaning* is characterized by mournful or murmuring sounds, wails, or laments in much louder than usual

volume. Loud groaning is characterized by louder than usual inarticulate, involuntary sounds, often abruptly beginning and ending.

6. *Crying* is characterized by an utterance of emotion accompanied by tears. There may be sobbing or quiet weeping.

## Facial Expression

1. *Smiling or inexpressive* is characterized by either upturned corners of the mouth, brightening of the eyes, and a look of pleasure or contentment or a neutral, at-ease, relaxed, or blank look.

2. *Sad* is characterized by an unhappy, lonesome, sorrowful, or dejected look. There may be tears in the eyes.

3. *Frightened* is characterized by a look of fear, alarm, or heightened anxiety. Eyes appear wide open.

4. *Frown* is characterized by a downward turn of the corners of the mouth. Increased facial wrinkling in the forehead and around the mouth may appear.

5. *Facial grimacing* is characterized by a distorted, distressed look. The brow is more wrinkled, as is the area around the mouth. Eyes may be squeezed shut.

## Body Language

1. *Relaxed* is characterized by a calm, restful, mellow appearance. The person seems to be taking it easy.

2. *Tense* is characterized by a strained, apprehensive, or worried appearance. The jaw may be clenched (exclude any contractures).

3. *Distressed pacing* is characterized by activity that seems unsettled. There may be a fearful, worried, or disturbed element present. The rate of walking may by faster or slower.

4. *Fidgeting* is characterized by restless movement. Squirming about or wiggling in the chair or bed may occur. The person might be hitching a chair across the room. Repetitive touching, tugging, or rubbing of body parts can also be observed.

5. *Rigid* is characterized by stiffening of the body. The arms and/ or legs are tight and inflexible. The trunk may appear straight and unyielding (exclude any contractures).

6. *Clenched fists* are characterized by tightly closed hands. They may be opened and closed repeatedly or held tightly shut.

7. *Knees pulled up* is characterized by flexing the legs and drawing the knees up toward the chest. May occur with an overall troubled appearance (exclude any contractures).

8. *Pulling or pushing away* is characterized by resistiveness upon approach or to care. The person is trying to escape by yanking or wrenching him- or herself free or by shoving the caregiver away.

9. *Striking out* is characterized by hitting, kicking, grabbing, punching, biting, or other forms of personal assault.

Consolability

1. *No need to console* is characterized by a sense of well-being. The person appears content.

2. *Distracted or reassured by voice or touch* is characterized by a disruption in the distressed behavior when the person is spoken to or touched. The behavior stops during the period of interaction, with no further indication that the person is distressed.

3. *Unable to console, distract, or reassure* is characterized by the inability to sooth the person or stop a behavior with words or actions. No amount of comforting—verbal or physical—will alleviate the behavior.

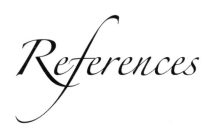

# References

Alzheimer's Association. (2005). *Dementia care practice recommendations for assisted living residences and nursing homes.* Chicago: Alzheimer's Association.

Alzheimer's Association. (2012a). *About us.* Retrieved from http://www.alz.org/about_us.asp

Alzheimer's Association. (2012b). *Alzheimer's disease facts and figures.* Retrieved from http://www.alz.org/downloads/facts_figures_2012.pdfme 8, Issue 2.

Alzheimer's Association. (2012c). *Brain health.* Retrieved from http://www.alz.org/we_can_help_brain_health_maintain_your_brain.asp

Asplund, K., Norberg, A., & Adolfsson, R. (1991). The sucking behaviour of two patients in the final stage of dementia of the Alzheimer type. *Scandinavian Journal of Caring Sciences, 5*(3), 141–147.

Bell, V., & Troxel, D. (1996, 2003). *The Best Friends approach to Alzheimer's care.* Baltimore: Health Professions Press.

Berman, B.M., Lao, L., Langenberg, P., Lee, W.L., Gilpin, A.M., & Hochberg, M.C. (2004). Effectiveness of acupuncture as adjunctive therapy in osteoarthritis of the knee: A randomized controlled trial. *Annals of Internal Medicine, 141*, 901–910.

Brawley, E.C. (1997). *Designing for Alzheimer's disease: Strategies for creating better care environments.* New York: Wiley.

Brawley, E.C. (2006). *Designing innovations for aging and Alzheimer's.* New York: Wiley.

Calkins, M.P. (2003). Research impacting design impacting research. *Alzheimer's Care Quarterly, 4*, 172–176.

Calkins, M.P. (2005). Environments for late-stage dementia. *Alzheimer's Care Quarterly, 6*, 71–75.

Calkins, M.P. (2009). Evidence-based long-term care design. *Neuro Rehabilitation, 25*(3), 145–154.

Callahan, S. (2005). Spiritual connections. *Alzheimer's Care Quarterly, 6*, 4–13.

Campbell-Taylor, I. (2008). Oropharyngeal dysphagia in long-term care: Misperception of treatment efficacy. *JAMA, 9*, 523–531.

Centers for Medicare & Medicaid Services (CMS). (2012). Nursing home quality initiative. Retrieved from http://www.cms.hhs.gov/NursingHomeQualityInits

Cuddy, L.L., & Duffin, J. (2005). Music, memory, and Alzheimer's disease: Is music recognition spared in dementia, and how can it be assessed? *Medical Hypotheses, 64,* 229–235.

Decker, F.H., Gruhn, P., Matthews-Martin, L., Dollard, K., Tucker, A., & Bizette, L. (2006). 2002 AHCA survey of nursing staff vacancy and turnover in nursing homes. Retrieved from http://www.ahcancal.org/research_data/staffing/Documents/Vacancy_Turnover_Survey2002.pdf

Dignity in Dying. (2008). Retrieved from http://www.dignityindying.org.uk/news/general/n41-survey-finds-that-being-alone-is-britains-biggest-fear-about-death

Feil, N. (1982). *V/F Validation: The Feil method.* Cleveland: Edward Feil Productions.

Feil, N. (2002). *The validation breakthrough* (2nd ed.). Baltimore: Health Professions Press.

Finucane, T.E., Christmas, C., & Travis, K. (1999). Tube feeding in patients with advanced dementia: A review of the evidence. *Journal of the American Medical Association, 282,* 1365–1370.

Flanagan, N. (1995). Essential oils and aromatherapy for Alzheimer's patients. *Alternative & Complementary Therapies,* 377–380.

Franssen, E.H., Reisberg, B., Kluger, A., Sinaiko, E., & Boja, C. (1991). Cognition-independent neurologic symptoms in normal aging and probable Alzheimer's disease. *Archives of Neurology, 2,* 148–154.

Fried, T.R., Gillick, M.R., & Lipsitz, L.A. (1995). Whether to transfer? Factors associated with hospitalization and outcome of elderly long-term care patients with pneumonia. *Journal of General Internal Medicine, 10,* 246–250.

Ghusan, H.F., Teasdale, T.A., Pepe, P.E., & Ginger, V.F. (1995). Older nursing home residents have a cardiac arrest survival rate similar to that of older persons living in the community. *Journal of the American Geriatrics Society, 43,* 520–527.

Gillick, M.R., & Mitchell, S.L. (2002). Facing eating difficulties in end-stage dementia. *Alzheimer's Care Quarterly, 3,* 227–232.

Goldschmidt, B., & van Meines, N. (2012). *Comforting touch in dementia and end of life care: Take my hand.* London: Jessica Kingsley Publishers.

The Green House Project. (2012). Frequently asked questions. Retrieved from http://thegreenhouseproject.org/about-us/frequently-asked-questions/

Hammar, L.M., Emami, A., Götell, E., & Engström, G. (2011). The impact of caregivers' singing on expressions of emotion and resistance during morning care situations in persons with dementia: An intervention in dementia care. *Journal of Clinical Nursing, 20,* 969–978.

Hellen, C.R. (1997). Communications and fundamentals of care: Bathing, grooming, and dressing. In C.R. Kovach (Ed.), *Late-stage dementia care: A basic guide* (pp. 113–125). Washington, DC: Taylor & Francis.

Holmes, C., Hopkins, V., Hensford, C., MacLaughlin, V., Wilkinson, D., & Rosenvinge, H. (2002). Lavender oil as a treatment for agitated behaviour in severe dementia: A placebo controlled study. *International Journal of Geriatric Psychiatry, 17*, 305–308.

Huffman, J.C., & Kunik, M.E. (2000). Assessment and understanding of pain in patients with dementia. *Gerontologist, 40*, 574–581.

International Center for Reiki Training. (2012). What is Reiki? Retrieved from http://www.reiki.org/faq/whatisreiki.html

Kessler, D. (1997). *The rights of the dying*. New York: HarperCollins.

Kitwood, T. (1998). Toward a theory of dementia care: Ethics and interaction. *Journal of Clinical Ethics, 9*, 23–34.

Kübler-Ross, E. (1969). *On death and dying*. New York: Macmillan.

Lin, P.W., Chan, W., Ng, B.F., & Lam, L.C. (2007). Efficacy of aromatherapy *(Lavandula angustifolia)* as an intervention for agitated behaviors in Chinese older persons with dementia: A cross-over randomized trial. *International Journal of Geriatric Psychiatry, 22*, 405–410.

Maurer, K., Volk, S., & Gerbaldo, H. (1997). Auguste D and Alzheimer's disease. *Lancet, 349*, 1546–1549.

Maxwell, T.I., et al. (2008). *UNIPAC One: The hospice and palliative medicine approach to life-limiting illness* (3rd ed.). New Rochelle, NY: Mary Ann Liebert.

Mehta, Z., Giorgini, K., Ellison, N., & Roth, M.E. (2012, March/April). Integrating palliative medicine with dementia care. *Aging Well*, pp. 18–20.

MetLife Foundation. (2011a). *Market survey of long-term care costs: The 2011 MetLife Market Survey of Nursing Home, Assisted Living, Adult Day Services, and Home Care Costs*. Retrieved from http://www.metlife.com/assets/cao/mmi/publications/studies/2011/mmi-market-survey-nursing-home-assisted-living-adult-day-services-costs.pdf

MetLife Foundation. (2011b). *What America thinks: MetLife Foundation Alzheimer's Survey*. Retrieved from http://www.metlife.com/assets/cao/contributions/foundation/alzheimers-2011.pdf

Miller, L., & Talerico, K.A. (2005). Development of an intervention to reduce pain in older adults with dementia. *Alzheimer's Care Quarterly, 6*, 154–167.

Mitchell, S.L., Teno, J.M., Miller, S.C., & Mor, V. (2005). A national study of the location of death for older persons with dementia. *Journal of the American Geriatrics Society, 53*, 299–305.

Morrison, R.S., Ahronheim, J.C., Morrison, G.R., Darling, E., Baskin, S.A., Morris, J., et al. (1998). Pain and discomfort associated with common hospital procedures and experiences. *Journal of Pain and Symptom Management, 15*, 91–101.

National Consensus Project. (2009). National Consensus Project for Quality Palliative Care. *Clinical Practice Guidelines for Quality Palliative Care*. Pittsburgh, PA.

National Hospice and Palliative Care Organization. (2012). Hospice care in America. Retrieved from http://www.nhpco.org/sites/default/files/public/Statistics_Research/2012_Facts_Figures.pdf

Orr-Rainey, N. (1994). The evolution of special care units: The nursing home industry perspective. *Journal of Alzheimer's Disease and Associated Disorders, 8*, 139–143.

Orsulic-Jeras, S., Judge, K.S., & Camp, C.J. (2000). Montessori-based activities for long-term care residents with advanced dementia: Effects on engagement and affect. *Gerontologist, 40*, 107–111.

Patient Self-Determination Act, P.L. 101-508, 42 U.S.C. § 1395 & 4751.

Simard, J. (2000). The Memory Enhancement Program: A new approach to increasing the quality of life for people with mild memory loss. In S.M. Albert (Ed.), *Assessing quality of life in Alzheimer's disease* (pp. 153–162). New York: Springer.

Simard, J. (2005). Namaste Care: Giving life to the end of life. *Alzheimer's Care Quarterly, 6*, 14–19.

Simard, J. (2007a). *The magic tape recorder*. Prague, Czech Republic: The Czech Alzheimer's Society.

Simard, J. (2007b). Silent and invisible: Nursing home residents with advanced dementia. *The Journal of Nutrition, Health & Aging, 6*(11), 484–488.

Simard, J. (2010). *Prague musings: Adventures & misadventures of an American living in Prague*. Joycesimard.com.

Simard, J. (2012a). One small miracle. *Journal of Gerontological Nursing, 38*(9), 52–56.

Simard, J. (2012b). Three little words. *Australian Journal of Dementia Care, 1*(3), 19–21.

Simard, J., & Volicer, L. (2002). The Club: Increasing the quality of life in dementia care. *Neurobiology of Aging, 23*, S540.

Simard, J., & Volicer, L. (2009). Management of advanced dementia. In M.F. Weiner & A.M. Lipton (Eds.), *Textbook of Alzheimer's Disease and Other Dementias*. Arlington, VA: The American Psychiatric Publishing (pp. 333–349).

Simard, J., & Volicer, L. (2010). Effects of Namaste Care on residents who do not benefit from usual activities. *American Journal of Alzheimer's Disease and Other Dementias, 25*, 46–50.

Smith, S.J. (1998). Providing palliative care for the terminal Alzheimer patient. In L. Volicer & A. Hurley (Eds.), *Hospice care for patients with advanced progressive dementia* (pp. 247–256). New York: Springer.

Spann, P. (2010). End-of-life care for patients with dementia. New York Times blog, The New Old Age. Retrieved from http://newoldage.blogs.nytimes.com/2010/11/02/end-of-life-care-for-patients-with-advanced-dementia/

Taylor, R. (2007). *Alzheimer's from the inside out*. Baltimore: Health Professions Press.

Thomas, W.H. (2004). *The Eden Alternative handbook*. Wimberley, TX: The Eden Alternative.

Volicer, L. (2005). End-of-life care for people with dementia in residential care settings. Alzheimer's Association. Retrieved from http://www.alz.org/national/documents/endoflifelitreview.pdf

Volicer, L. (2007). Terminal stage. In S. Gauthier (Ed.), *Clinical diagnosis and management of Alzheimer's disease* (3rd ed., pp. 247–255). Oxon, England: Informa Healthcare.

Volicer, L. (2012). Palliative care in dementia. *Palliative Care Journal.* In press.

Volicer, L., Cantor, M.D., Derse, A.R., Edwards, D.M., Prudhomme, A.M., Gregory, D.C., et al. (2002). Advanced care planning by proxy for residents of long-term care facilities who lack decision-making capacity. *Journal of the American Geriatric Society, 50,* 761–767.

Volicer, L., McKee, A., & Hewitt, S. (2001). Dementia. *Neurologic Clinics of North America, 19,* 867–885.

Volicer, L., Simard, J., Pupa, J.H., Medrek, R., & Riordan, M.E. (2006). Effect of continuous activity programming on behavioral symptoms of dementia. *Journal of the American Medical Directors Association, 7,* 426–431.

Warden, V., Hurley, A.C., & Volicer, L. (2003). Development and psychometric evaluation of the PAINAD (Pain Assessment in Advanced Dementia) Scale. *Journal of the American Medical Directors Association, 4,* 9–15.

Williams, C.S., Zimmerman, S., Sloane, P.D., Reed, P.S. (2005). Characteristics associated with pain in long-term care residents with dementia. *Gerontologist, 45*(1), 68–73.

# Index

Note: *b* indicates boxes.